Sexual Respect Guide

Guía de Respeto Sexual

دليل الاحترام الجنسي

I0426893

By

Marisa L. Williams

Sexual Respect Guide

Guía de Respeto Sexual

دليل الاحترام الجنسي

By

Marisa L. Williams

ISBN: 978-1-387-75892-0
Imprint: Lulu.com

Covering Relationship Basics

Cubriendo los conceptos básicos de la relación

تغطية أساسيات العلاقة

Don't Be Scared

No te asustes

لا تخف

Don't be scared to start a conversation. The days of cheesy pickup lines in hazy, smoke-filled bars are over; although, asking for a lighter is one way to start a conversation. No matter if it's talking about the weather, a news story or whatever you come up with, if you don't know where to start, compliments are always welcome, so long as they are not vulgar.

Does something in their outfit catch your eye? Be genuine, and the more innocent, the better, such as complimenting a piece of jewelry or other accessory in their outfit, even socks. Even if you drop a small compliment in passing, and go in for a deeper conversation later, it serves as a great ice breaker and makes the person feel better about themselves simultaneously.

This does not mean saying, "hey, nice ass!" That's too much. Subtle is smooth.

No tengas miedo de iniciar una conversación. Los días de las líneas de recolección cursis en bares brumosos y llenos de humo han terminado; aunque, pedir un encendedor es una forma de iniciar una conversación. No importa si se trata del clima, una noticia o lo que se te ocurra, si no sabes por dónde empezar, los cumplidos siempre son bienvenidos, siempre y cuando no sean vulgares.

¿Te llama la atención algo en su atuendo? Sea genuino, y cuanto más inocente, mejor, como complementar una pieza de joyería u otro accesorio en su atuendo, incluso calcetines. Incluso si dejas caer un pequeño cumplido de pasada y entras en una conversación más profunda más tarde, sirve como un gran rompehielos y hace que la persona se sienta mejor consigo misma simultáneamente.

Esto no significa decir: "¡oye, buen culo!" Eso es demasiado. Sutil es suave.

لا تخف من بدء محادثة. لقد ولت أيام خطوط الالتقاط الجبنة في الحانات الضبابية المليئة بالدخان. على الرغم من أن طلب ولاعة هو إحدى الطرق لبدء محادثة. بغض النظر عما إذا كان يتحدث عن الطقس أو قصة إخبارية أو أي شيء تتوصل إليه ، إذا كنت لا تعرف من أين تبدأ ، فإن المجاملات مرحب بها دائما ، طالما أنها ليست مبتذلة.

هل هناك شيء ما في ملابسهم يلفت انتباهك؟ كن صادقا ، وكلما كانت أكثر براءة ، كان ذلك أفضل ، مثل مجاملة قطعة من المجوهرات أو غيرها من الملحقات في ملابسهم ، حتى الجوارب. حتى لو أسقطت مجاملة صغيرة عابرة ، وذهبت

لإجراء محادثة أعمق لاحقا ، فإنها بمثابة كاسحة جليد رائعة
وتجعل الشخص يشعر بتحسن تجاه نفسه في وقت واحد.

هذا لا يعني القول ،"مهلا ، الحمار لطيف "! هذا
أكثر من اللازم. خفية على نحو سلس.

Don't Be Grabby

No te quedes agarrado

لا تكن مغرما

Once engaged in conversation and while entering their space, do not be overly grabby or aggressive. A forceful grab of the wrist is enough to turn someone's internal alarm on warning. Instead, be nice, remain calm, do not act as if this is the last person you will ever see on Earth.

Leaving bruises is never a good thing, as that can be enough to alert authorities. Avoid unwanted attention, and if someone says no, do not press the issue a million times to make them cave into something they already told you they do not want to do. Never high pressure.

If someone wants to be kinky in the bedroom, that's an entirely different topic. For a first meeting, don't grab someone or rub your genitals on *them in an inappropriate manner. Do not try to feel up someone's private parts upon a first meeting in an unwanted manner either.*

Una vez que participe en la conversación y al entrar en su espacio, no sea demasiado agarrado o agresivo. Un agarre contundente de la muñeca es suficiente para activar la alarma interna de alguien en advertencia. En cambio, sé amable, mantén la calma, no actúes como si esta fuera la última persona que verás en la Tierra.

Dejar moretones nunca es algo bueno, ya que eso puede ser suficiente para alertar a las autoridades. Evita la atención no deseada, y si alguien dice que no, no presiones el tema un millón de veces para que cedan en algo que ya te dijeron que no quieren hacer. Nunca alta presión.

Si alguien quiere ser pervertido en el dormitorio, ese es un tema completamente diferente. Para una primera reunión, no agarres a alguien ni frotes tus genitales sobre ellos de manera inapropiada. Tampoco trates de sentir las partes íntimas de alguien en una primera reunión de una manera no deseada.

بمجرد الانخراط في محادثة وأثناء دخول مساحتهم ، لا تكن ممسكا أو عدوانيا بشكل مفرط. إن الإمساك القوي بالمعصم

يكفي لتشغيل التنبيه الداخلي لشخص ما عند التحذير. بدلا من ذلك ، كن لطيفا ، وابق هادئا ، ولا تتصرف كما لو كان هذا هو آخر شخص ستراه على الأرض.

ترك الكدمات ليس بالأمر الجيد أبدا ، لأن ذلك يمكن أن يكون كافيا لتنبيه السلطات. تجنب الاهتمام غير المرغوب فيه ، وإذا قال شخص ما لا ، فلا تضغط على المشكلة مليون مرة لجعله يستسلم لشيء أخبرك بالفعل أنه لا يريد القيام به. أبدا الضغط العالي.

إذا أراد شخص ما أن يكون غريبا في غرفة النوم ، فهذا موضوع مختلف تماما. في الاجتماع الأول، لا تمسك بشخص ما أو تفرك أعضائك التناسلية عليه بطريقة غير لائقة. لا تحاول أن تشعر بالأجزاء الخاصة لشخص ما عند الاجتماع الأول بطريقة غير مرغوب فيها أيضا.

Treat People Nice

Tratar a la gente bien

علاج الناس لطيفة

It's pretty basic. Treat as others as you would like them to treat you. If you yell and scream, expect someone to do the same thing back. If frustrations get high, peacefully take a momentary breather from each other and the situation, until both of you can resume calm talk.

There's no need to come to slaps, kicks, bites, punches or any type of adolescent behavior. If you cannot act like an adult, excuse yourself from the situation until you can. It takes to engage in an argument, so if one is not there, then the other can blow off steam.

This does not mean run away entirely. Sometimes, people will feel abandoned that way. It means simply go into another room, take a few minutes to compose yourself or as long as needed to be able to act like an adult, then try to solve any problems in a calm manner.

Es bastante básico. Trata como a los demás como te gustaría que te trataran a ti. Si gritas y gritas, espera que alguien haga lo mismo. Si las frustraciones se elevan, tome un respiro momentáneo el uno del otro y de la situación, hasta que ambos puedan reanudar la conversación tranquila.

No hay necesidad de llegar a bofetadas, patadas, mordeduras, puñetazos o cualquier tipo de comportamiento adolescente. Si no puedes actuar como un adulto, discúlpate de la situación hasta que puedas. Se necesita participar en una discusión, por lo que si uno no está allí, entonces el otro puede desahogarse.

Esto no significa huir por completo. A veces, las personas se sentirán abandonadas de esa manera.

Significa simplemente ir a otra habitación, tomarse unos minutos para componerse o el tiempo que sea necesario para poder actuar como un adulto, luego tratar de resolver cualquier problema de una manera tranquila.

انها بسيطة جدا .تعامل مع الآخرين كما تريد منهم أن يعاملوك .إذا كنت تصرخ وتصرخ ، فتوقع من شخص ما أن يفعل الشيء نفسه مرة أخرى .إذا ارتفعت الإحباطات ، خذ نفسا لحظيا من بعضكما البعض والموقف بسلام ، حتى يتمكن كلاكما من استئناف الحديث الهادئ.

ليست هناك حاجة للصفع أو الركلات أو اللدغات أو اللكمات أو أي نوع من سلوك المراهقين .إذا كنت لا تستطيع التصرف كشخص بالغ ، فاعذر نفسك من الموقف حتى تتمكن من ذلك .يتطلب الأمر الدخول في جدال ، لذلك إذا لم يكن أحدهما موجودا ، فيمكن للآخر أن ينفجر البخار.

هذا لا يعني الهروب تماما .في بعض الأحيان ، سيشعر الناس بأنهم مهجورون بهذه الطريقة .هذا يعني ببساطة الذهاب إلى غرفة أخرى ، ويستغرق بضع دقائق لتكوين نفسك أو طالما كان ذلك ضروريا لتكون قادرا على التصرف مثل شخص بالغ ، ثم حاول حل أي مشاكل بطريقة هادئة.

Respect Your Lover

Respeta a tu amante

احترم حبيبك

Do not talk down to your lover, as you are there to be a lover, not a hater. Never call your lover stupid or insignificant. Make them feel as if their opinion counts and matters.

People like to feel acknowledged. Leaving little love letters for them to find can be a great way to add some chemistry to the mix, as partners love knowing what you find attractive in them. They like knowing they please you, and you find them attractive as well, so tell them.

Take an interest in what they do. Make their accomplishments something you are proud of, congratulating them on a job well done, even if it's something as silly as frosting a cake. Sharing positive vibes with them only strengthens the connection and makes sex all the better.

No hables mal de tu amante, ya que estás ahí para ser un amante, no un odiador. Nunca llames a tu amante estúpido o insignificante. Hazles sentir que su opinión cuenta y importa.

A la gente le gusta sentirse reconocida. Dejar pequeñas cartas de amor para que las encuentren puede ser una excelente manera de agregar algo de química a la mezcla, ya que a las parejas les encanta saber lo que encuentras atractivo en ellas. Les gusta saber que te agradan, y tú también los encuentras atractivos, así que cuéntalos.

Interesarse por lo que hacen. Haz de sus logros algo de lo que estés orgulloso, felicitándolos por un trabajo bien hecho, incluso si es algo tan tonto como glasear un pastel. Compartir vibraciones positivas con ellos solo fortalece la conexión y hace que el sexo sea aún mejor.

لا تتحدث إلى حبيبك ، لأنك هناك لتكون حبيبا ، وليس كارها. لا تسمي حبيبك غبيا أو تافها. اجعلهم يشعرون كما لو أن رأيهم مهم ومهم.

يحب الناس أن يشعروا بالتقدير. يمكن أن يكون ترك رسائل حب صغيرة لهم للعثور عليها طريقة رائعة لإضافة بعض الكيمياء إلى المزيج ، حيث يحب الشركاء معرفة ما تجده جذابا فيهم. إنهم يحبون معرفة أنهم يرضونك وتجدهم جذابين أيضا ، لذا أخبرهم ،

اهتم بما يفعلونه. اجعل إنجازاتهم شيئا تفخر به ، وهنأهم على عمل جيد ، حتى لو كان شيئا سخيفا مثل صقيع الكعكة. مشاركة المشاعر الإيجابية معهم فقط يقوي الاتصال ويجعل الجنس أفضل.

No Superiority Complexes
Sin complejos de superioridad
لا توجد مجمعات تفوق

Nobody likes to feel lesser or unworthy, so don't act like you're better than your lover. Don't act like your opinion matters more, like you're smarter, and don't make them feel dumb. It's better to take the stance of a teacher who is willing to explain something than to make a lover feel like they're beneath you or too stupid to understand a topic.

Do not play the earn my affection game. If you feel that your lover must earn your affection, then either you're too controlling, or you're with the wrong lover. Affection should be given freely.

If you do not feel affectionate towards your lover, ask yourself why. Is it the wrong person, or are there simply hurt feelings that need to be cleared? Hold your partner up on a pedestal.

A nadie le gusta sentirse menos o indigno, así que no actúes como si fueras mejor que tu amante. No actúes como si tu opinión importara más, como si fueras más inteligente, y no los hagas sentir tontos.

Es mejor tomar la postura de un maestro que está dispuesto a explicar algo que hacer que un amante sienta que está debajo de ti o que es demasiado estúpido para entender un tema.

No juegues al juego de ganar mi afecto. Si sientes que tu amante debe ganarse tu afecto, entonces eres demasiado controlador o estás con el amante equivocado. El afecto debe darse libremente.

Si no te sientes cariñoso con tu amante, pregúntate por qué. ¿Es la persona equivocada, o simplemente hay sentimientos heridos que necesitan ser aclarados? Sostenga a su pareja en un pedestal.

لا أحد يحب أن يشعر بأنه أقل أو لا يستحق ، لذلك لا تتصرف وكأنك أفضل من حبيبك. لا تتصرف كما لو أن رأيك يهم أكثر ، كما لو كنت أكثر ذكاء ، ولا تجعلهم يشعرون بالغباء. من الأفضل أن تتخذ موقف المعلم المستعد لشرح شيء ما بدلا من جعل الحبيب يشعر وكأنه تحتك أو غبي جدا لفهم موضوع ما.

لا تلعب لعبة كسب عاطفتي. إذا كنت تشعر أن حبيبك يجب أن يكسب عاطفتك ، فإما أنك مسيطر للغاية ، أو أنك مع الحبيب الخطأ. يجب إعطاء المودة بحرية.

إذا كنت لا تشعر بالحنان تجاه حبيبك ، اسأل نفسك لماذا. هل هو الشخص الخطأ ، أم أن هناك ببساطة مشاعر جارحة تحتاج إلى تطهيرها؟ احمل شريكك على قاعدة التمثال.

Don't Mention Others

No menciones a los demás

لا تذكر الآخرين

An ex of mine had a rule not to mention members of the opposite sex, and that worked very well to reduce any jealous issues. It's hard to be jealous of someone if you don't know about them, as their name is never mentioned in the first place. If it is an ex, or someone you do not plan on your lover meeting, ask yourself how dire is it for your lover to hear that story?

Is it worth bringing up an ex and creating a potential jealousy issue? Would it be easier to simply not tell the story, even if you really want to? What will telling it help?

If you find the story may do more harm than good, or it is simply not necessary, then think twice about creating jealous issues by talking about an ex or another potential interest. Sure, we want our lover to know about us, but do they need to know everything from our past in the first five minutes of meeting, or can we listen to what they have to say and observe?

Un ex mío tenía una regla para no mencionar a los miembros del sexo opuesto, y eso funcionó muy bien para reducir cualquier problema de celos. Es difícil estar celoso de alguien si no lo conoces, ya que su nombre nunca se menciona en primer lugar. Si es un ex, o alguien que no planeas conocer con tu amante, pregúntate qué tan grave es para tu amante escuchar esa historia.

¿Vale la pena traer a un ex y crear un posible problema de celos? ¿Sería más fácil simplemente no contar la historia, incluso si realmente quieres? ¿Qué ayudará contarlo?

كان لدى شخص سابق لي قاعدة بعدم ذكر أعضاء الجنس الآخر ، وقد نجح ذلك بشكل جيد للغاية للحد من أي مشاكل غيورة. من الصعب أن تشعر بالغيرة من شخص ما إذا كنت لا تعرف عنه ، حيث لا يتم ذكر اسمه في المقام الأول. إذا كان شخصا سابقا ، أو شخصا لا تخطط للقاء حبيبك ، اسأل نفسك ما مدى صعوبة سماع حبيبك لهذه القصة؟

هل يستحق الأمر إثارة شخص سابق وخلق مشكلة غيرة محتملة ، ؟ هل سيكون من الأسهل ببساطة عدم سرد القصة حتى لو كنت تريد ذلك حقا؟ ما الذي سيساعدها؟

No Love Triangles

Sin triángulos amorosos

لا مثلثات الحب

Within the rule of not mentioning others includes talks of threesomes early in a budding relationship. Even if it has always been a fantasy, focus on pleasing one lover, and mastering the one person, before you are concerned about another. In most threesomes, someone is feeling left out, which can create feelings of jealous, which can erode relationships entirely.

Mentioning the desire for a threesome can make a lover feel as if they are not satisfying you enough on their own. If talks of fantasies comes up later, that's a different story, but if you are still getting to know someone, don't make them feel as if they do not satisfy you. This includes not mentioning specific people you fantasize about having a threesome with.

If a lover feels as if they cannot trust you around their friends, that's an issue. Don't create that issue by saying you want to have threesomes with their friends right off the bat. In fact, it's best to not mention fantasies about close acquaintances to prevent jealousy issues.

Dentro de la regla de no mencionar a los demás se incluyen las conversaciones de tríos al principio de una relación en ciernes. Incluso si siempre ha sido una fantasía, concéntrate en complacer a un amante y dominar a una persona, antes de preocuparte por otra. En la mayoría de los tríos, alguien se siente excluido, lo que puede crear sentimientos de celos, lo que puede erosionar las relaciones por completo.

Mencionar el deseo de un trío puede hacer que un amante se sienta como si no te estuviera satisfaciendo lo suficiente por sí solo. Si las conversaciones de fantasías surgen más tarde, esa es una historia diferente, pero si todavía estás conociendo a alguien, no lo hagas sentir como si no te satisficiera. Esto incluye no mencionar a personas específicas con las que fantaseas con tener un trío.

Si un amante siente que no puede confiar en ti alrededor de sus amigos, eso es un problema. No crees ese problema diciendo que quieres tener tríos con sus amigos de inmediato. De hecho, es mejor no mencionar las fantasías sobre conocidos cercanos para evitar problemas de celos.

ضمن قاعدة عدم ذكر الآخرين يتضمن محادثات عن الثلاثي في وقت مبكر من علاقة ناشئة. حتى لو كان الأمر دائما خيالا ، ركز على إرضاء حبيب واحد ، وإتقان شخص واحد

، قبل أن تشعر بالقلق إزاء شخص آخر .في معظم الثلاثي ،
، يشعر شخص ما بأنه مهمل ، مما قد يخلق مشاعر بالغيرة
.والتي يمكن أن تؤدي إلى تآكل العلاقات تماما

إن ذكر الرغبة في الثلاثي يمكن أن يجعل الحبيب
يشعر كما لو أنه لا يرضيك بما فيه الكفاية بمفرده .إذا
ظهرت محادثات عن الأوهام في وقت لاحق ، فهذه قصة
مختلفة ، ولكن إذا كنت لا تزال تتعرف على شخص ما ، فلا
تجعله يشعر كما لو أنه لا يرضيك .وهذا يشمل عدم ذكر
.أشخاص محددين تتخيل وجود ثلاثة أشخاص معهم

إذا شعر الحبيب كما لو أنه لا يستطيع الوثوق بك حول
أصدقائه ، فهذه مشكلة .لا تخلق هذه المشكلة بالقول إنك
تريد أن يكون لديك ثلاثة أشخاص مع أصدقائهم مباشرة من
الخفافيش .في الواقع ، من الأفضل عدم ذكر الأوهام حول
.المعارف المقربين لمنع مشكلات الغيرة

A Responsible Lover

Un amante responsable

عاشق مسؤول

*Especially if you do have other partners, be a
responsible lover and get checked regularly for sexual
diseases. The three-week rule that is takes about
three weeks for many sexual diseases and pregnancy
to be detected accurately. Wait three weeks after a
new partner, then get tested, as if you go the day*

after hooking up with someone, it may not detect problems yet.

Take responsibility for your own actions. Own up to things you did that may have hurt your lover, and do not try to spin the tables or deflect. Solve the problem and move on.

Be open and honest, but don't try to be mean, spiteful and hurtful. Censor those things when you can. Try to bring the positive at all times, as negative emotions spill over to others.

Especialmente si tiene otras parejas, sea un amante responsable y hágase revisar regularmente para detectar enfermedades sexuales. La regla de las tres semanas que toma alrededor de tres semanas para que muchas enfermedades sexuales y el embarazo se detecten con precisión. Espere tres semanas después de una nueva pareja, luego hágase la prueba, ya que si va al día siguiente de conectarse con alguien, es posible que aún no detecte problemas.

Asume la responsabilidad de tus propias acciones. Reconozca las cosas que hizo que pueden haber lastimado a su amante, y no trate de girar las mesas o desviarse. Resuelve el problema y sigue adelante.

Sé abierto y honesto, pero no trates de ser malo, rencoroso e hiriente. Censura esas cosas cuando puedas. Trate de traer lo positivo en todo

momento, ya que las emociones negativas se
extienden a los demás.

خاصة إذا كان لديك شركاء آخرون ، كن عاشقا مسؤولا
وتحقق بانتظام من الأمراض الجنسية .قاعدة الأسابيع
الثلاثة التي تستغرق حوالي ثلاثة أسابيع حتى يتم اكتشاف
العديد من الأمراض الجنسية والحمل بدقة .انتظر ثلاثة
أسابيع بعد شريك جديد ، ثم قم بالاختبار ، كما لو كنت تذهب
في اليوم التالي للارتباط بشخص ما ، فقد لا يكتشف المشاكل
بعد.

تحمل المسؤولية عن أفعالك الخاصة .امتلك الأشياء
التي قمت بها والتي قد تكون قد آذت حبيبك ، ولا تحاول
تدوير الطاولات أو الانحراف .حل المشكلة والمضي قدما.

كن منفتحا وصادقا ، لكن لا تحاول أن تكون حقيرا
وحاقدا ومؤذيا .فرض رقابة على هذه الأشياء عندما
تستطيع .حاول أن تجلب الإيجابية في جميع الأوقات ، حيث
تمتد المشاعر السلبية إلى الآخرين.

No one-way

No hay unidireccional

لا يوجد اتجاه واحد

A relationship cannot be one-way. Meaning, it should be give and take. Not just one person taking.

Una relación no puede ser unidireccional. Es decir, debe ser dar y recibir. No solo una persona tomando.

لا يمكن أن تكون العلاقة في اتجاه واحد .بمعنى ، يجب أن يكون الأخذ والعطاء .ليس فقط شخص واحد يأخذ.

Even if it is a sugar baby situation, there is a duty to make a lover feel as if they are getting something back in return for whatever type of relationship status. If one person continually gives, and another continually takes, the situation will grow tiresome after too long. Always be sure there is at least a little give and take from both parties, as it's the push and pull that balances.

Incluso si se trata de una situación de sugar baby, existe el deber de hacer que un amante se sienta como si estuviera recibiendo algo a cambio de cualquier tipo de estado de relación. Si una persona da continuamente, y otra toma continuamente, la situación se volverá agotadora después de demasiado tiempo. Siempre asegúrese de que haya al menos un poco de toma y daca de ambas partes, ya que es el empuje y el tirón lo que se equilibra.

حتى لو كان الأمر يتعلق بطفل السكر ، فهناك واجب لجعل الحبيب يشعر كما لو أنه يحصل على شيء ما مقابل أي نوع من حالة العلاقة .إذا أعطى شخص ما باستمرار ، وأخذ آخر

باستمرار ، فإن الوضع سيزداد إرهاقا بعد فترة طويلة جدا.
تأكد دائما من وجود القليل من الأخذ والعطاء على الأقل من
كلا الطرفين ، لأن الدفع والسحب هو الذي يوازن.

Just like with yoga stretching, sometimes pushing in the opposite direction will deepen a stretch. It's the same with relationships. Too much of one direction for too long does not work and will result in the opposite.

Al igual que con el estiramiento de yoga, a veces empujar en la dirección opuesta profundizará un estiramiento. Es lo mismo con las relaciones. Demasiado de una dirección durante demasiado tiempo no funciona y resultará en lo contrario.

تماما كما هو الحال مع اليوغا تمتد ، في بعض الأحيان دفع
في الاتجاه المعاكس سوف يعمق التمدد. الأمر نفسه مع
العلاقات. الكثير من اتجاه واحد لفترة طويلة جدا لا يعمل
وسوف يؤدي إلى عكس ذلك.

Supportively Suggest Change

Sugerir un cambio de apoyo

اقتراح التغيير بشكل داعم

If there's something you want to suggest changing about your lover, do not be mean about it.

Don't say, "hey, Fat Ass, you need to lose some weight you tub of lard!" That will not produce the desired effect, so try suggesting activities that might produce the effect that you can help be a positive and supporting partner, such as a couples walk each evening.

Instead of saying, "your lazy ass needs to get a job," you can simply ask your partner where they would desire to work. What are their interests, and how can they make money from those interests? Try to open a supportive dialogue that makes them feel valued.

Sometimes, people need help taking that first step towards action, and if you can help inspire them, that is much better than talking down to anyone. Partners should be supportive of each other, and breaking bad habits can be hard, but it's not impossible with creativity.

Si hay algo que quieres sugerir cambiar sobre tu amante, no seas malo al respecto. No digas: ¡Oye, Gordo, necesitas perder algo de peso en tu tina de manteca de cerdo! Eso no producirá el efecto deseado, así que trate de sugerir actividades que puedan producir el efecto de que puede ayudar a ser un compañero positivo y de apoyo, como una caminata de pareja cada noche.

En lugar de decir: tu perezoso necesita conseguir un trabajo, simplemente puedes preguntarle a tu pareja dónde desearía trabajar. ¿Cuáles son sus intereses y cómo pueden ganar dinero con esos intereses? Trate de abrir un diálogo de apoyo que los haga sentir valorados.

A veces, las personas necesitan ayuda para dar ese primer paso hacia la acción, y si puedes ayudar a inspirarlos, eso es mucho mejor que hablar mal de nadie. Las parejas deben apoyarse mutuamente, y romper los malos hábitos puede ser difícil, pero no es imposible con la creatividad.

إذا كان هناك شيء تريد اقتراح تغييره عن حبيبك ، فلا تكن وقحا بشأنه . لا تقل ، "مهلا ، الحمار الدهني ، تحتاج إلى فقدان بعض الوزن الذي تتناوله في حوض شحم الخنزير!" لن ينتج عن ذلك التأثير المطلوب ، لذا حاول اقتراح الأنشطة التي قد تنتج التأثير الذي يمكنك من خلاله المساعدة في أن تكون شريكا إيجابيا وداعما ، مثل المشي بين الأزواج كل مساء.

بدلا من قول "يحتاج مؤخرتك الكسولة إلى الحصول على وظيفة" ، يمكنك ببساطة أن تسأل شريكك عن المكان الذي يرغب في العمل فيه . ما هي مصالحهم، وكيف يمكنهم كسب المال من تلك المصالح؟ حاول فتح حوار داعم يجعلهم يشعرون بالتقدير.

في بعض الأحيان ، يحتاج الناس إلى المساعدة في اتخاذ هذه الخطوة الأولى نحو العمل ، وإذا كان بإمكانك المساعدة في

إلهامهم ، فهذا أفضل بكثير من التحدث إلى أي شخص يجب
أن يكون الشركاء داعمين لبعضهم البعض ، وقد يكون كسر
العادات السيئة أمرا صعبا ، لكنه ليس مستحيلا مع الإبداع.

Acknowledge Your Lover

Reconoce a tu amante

اعترف بحبيبك

Never make your lover feel as if they are not part of the party. Don't make a lover feel as if they need to keep quiet in the back, while you have all the fun. Make your lover part of the activities to make them feel as if they are a part of your life, valued and appreciated.

Introduce them to your friends and family. Make them feel as if they are an important part of your life. Do not make them feel as if you are ashamed of them or keeping them hidden.

Say hello, goodbye, good morning and good night to each other. Communicate regularly and effectively. Ask what your lover likes to do, watch or listen to, so it's not all about you.

Nunca hagas que tu amante se sienta como si no fuera parte de la fiesta. No hagas que un amante se sienta como si necesitara guardar silencio en la parte de atrás, mientras tú te diviertes. Haz que tu amante forme parte de las actividades para que se sienta parte de tu vida, valorado y apreciado.

Preséntalos a tus amigos y familiares. Haz que se sientan como si fueran una parte importante de tu vida. No los hagas sentir como si estuvieras avergonzado de ellos o manteniéndolos ocultos.

Saluda, adiós, buenos días y buenas noches el uno al otro. Comunícate de manera regular y efectiva. Pregúntale a tu amante qué le gusta hacer, ver o escuchar, para que no todo se trate de ti.

لا تجعل حبيبك يشعر كما لو أنه ليس جزءا من الحفلة. لا تجعل الحبيب يشعر كما لو كان بحاجة إلى التزام الصمت في الخلف ، بينما لديك كل المتعة. اجعل حبيبك جزءا من الأنشطة لجعله يشعر كما لو كان جزءا من حياتك ، ويقدر ويقدر.

قدمهم إلى أصدقائك وعائلتك. اجعلهم يشعرون كما لو كانوا جزءا مهما من حياتك. لا تجعلهم يشعرون كما لو كنت تخجل منهم أو تبقيهم مختبئين.

قل مرحبا ، وداعا ، صباح الخير وليلة سعيدة لبعضنا البعض. التواصل بانتظام وفعالية. اسأل عما يحب حبيبك القيام به أو مشاهدته أو الاستماع إليه ، لذلك ليس كل شيء عنك.

Have Date Nights

Tener citas nocturnas

هل لديك ليالي التاريخ

Have regularly scheduled dates. Experience things together. Bond.

Don't be like passing ships in the night where you barely see each other. Make time to spend with each other at least every other week. Coordinate mutual days off and have fun.

Spending time together, taking a break from the normal grind, can be as innocent as getting an ice cream cone or taking a walk through a park. It does not have to be extravagant. Sometimes simple things allow for more time talking with each other about each other's lives.

Tener fechas programadas regularmente. Experimenten las cosas juntos. Vinculación.

No seas como pasar barcos en la noche donde apenas se ven. Tómese el tiempo para pasar juntos al menos cada dos semanas. Coordina los días libres mutuos y diviértete.

Pasar tiempo juntos, tomar un descanso de la rutina normal, puede ser tan inocente como conseguir un cono de helado o dar un paseo por un parque. No tiene por qué ser extravagante. A veces, las cosas simples permiten más tiempo hablando entre sí sobre la vida del otro.

لديك تواريخ مجدولة بانتظام. اختبر الأشياء معا. السندات.

لا تكن مثل السفن المارة في الليل حيث بالكاد ترى بعضكما البعض. خصص وقتا لقضاء الوقت مع بعضهم البعض على الأقل كل أسبوعين. تنسيق أيام العطلة المتبادلة والمتعة.

يمكن أن يكون قضاء بعض الوقت معا ، وأخذ استراحة من الطحن العادي ، بريئا مثل الحصول على مخروط الآيس كريم أو المشي في الحديقة. ليس من الضروري أن تكون باهظة. في بعض الأحيان تسمح الأشياء البسيطة بمزيد من الوقت للتحدث مع بعضهم البعض حول حياة بعضهم البعض.

Gift Each Other

Regalarse unos a otros

إهداء بعضنا البعض

Give gifts generously. They do not have to be expensive. They can be free compliments.

Tell your lover when they look nice. Pick a flower to give to them. Draw them a heart in the sand or the snow with both of your initials in it as if you were still school-aged.

Give what you can when you can to let your lover know you are thinking of them. A love note scribbled on a napkin can be just as generous as something more expensive. It's the thought that counts, showing them that they are in your thoughts on a regular basis.

Da regalos generosamente. No tienen por qué ser caros. Pueden ser cumplidos gratuitos.

Dígale a su amante cuando se vea bien. Elige una flor para dársela. Dibuja un corazón en la arena o la nieve con tus dos iniciales como si todavía estuvieras en edad escolar.

Da lo que puedas cuando puedas para que tu amante sepa que estás pensando en ellos. Una nota de amor garabateada en una servilleta puede ser tan generosa como algo más caro. Es el pensamiento lo que cuenta, mostrándoles que están en tus pensamientos de forma regular.

قدم الهدايا بسخاء .ليس من الضروري أن تكون باهظة الثمن .يمكن أن تكون مجاملات مجانية

أخبر حبيبك عندما تبدو لطيفة .اختر زهرة لإعطائها لهم .ارسم لهم قلبا في الرمال أو الثلج مع كل من الأحرف الأولى من اسمك فيه كما لو كنت لا تزال في سن المدرسة.

أعط ما تستطيع عندما تستطيع أن تدع حبيبك يعرف أنك تفكر فيه .يمكن أن تكون مذكرة الحب المخربشة على منديل سخية مثل شيء أكثر تكلفة .إنها الفكرة التي تهم ، وتبين لهم أنهم في أفكارك على أساس منتظم.

Do Not Accuse

No acusar

لا تتهم

The French have a saying: "the man does not look behind the door, unless the man has stood there once before." In other words, we are often guilty of accusing people of doing things that we have done ourselves at some point. Let's not deflect our pasts onto our partners.

Trauma runs deep. Once we get hurt, we worry we will be hurt again. Accusations can be blurted out of fear, and while not knowing creates anxiety, avoid drama by not accusing people of stuff they likely did not really do, and save confrontation until you have solid facts.

Randomly accusing people of things only lets them know that you do not trust them. As good relationships should be built on trust and mutual respect, pointing the finger of blame when you don't know for sure only creates unnecessary drama, so investigate thoroughly. When you have your facts in a row, you can calmly discuss whatever you may have discovered.

Los franceses tienen un dicho: "el hombre no mira detrás de la puerta, a menos que el hombre se haya parado allí una vez antes". En otras palabras, a menudo somos culpables de acusar a las personas de hacer cosas que nosotros mismos hemos hecho en algún momento. No desviemos nuestro pasado hacia nuestros socios.

El trauma es profundo. Una vez que nos lastimamos, nos preocupa que volvamos a ser lastimados. Las acusaciones se pueden soltar por miedo, y aunque no saber crea ansiedad, evite el drama al no acusar a las personas de cosas que probablemente no hicieron realmente, y evite la confrontación hasta que tenga hechos sólidos.

Acusar al azar a las personas de cosas solo les hace saber que no confías en ellas. Como las buenas relaciones deben construirse sobre la confianza y el respeto mutuo, señalar con el dedo acusador cuando no lo sabes con certeza solo crea un drama innecesario, así que investiga a fondo. Cuando tenga sus hechos seguidos, puede discutir con calma lo que haya descubierto.

لدى الفرنسيين قول مأثور" :الرجل لا ينظر خلف الباب ، إلا إذا كان الرجل قد وقف هناك مرة واحدة من قبل »بعبارة أخرى، غالبا ما نكون مذنبين باتهام الناس بالقيام بأشياء فعلناها بأنفسنا في مرحلة ما .دعونا لا نحرف ماضينا إلى شركائنا.

الصدمة عميقة .بمجرد أن نتأذى ، نشعر بالقلق من أننا سنتعرض للأذى مرة أخرى .يمكن طمس الاتهامات بدافع الخوف ، وبينما يؤدي عدم المعرفة إلى خلق القلق ، تجنب الدراما من خلال عدم اتهام الناس بأشياء من المحتمل أنهم لم يفعلوها حقا ، وحفظ المواجهة حتى يكون لديك حقائق صلبة.

إن اتهام الناس عشوائيا بالأشياء يتيح لهم فقط معرفة أنك لا تثق بهم .نظرا لأن العلاقات الجيدة يجب أن تبنى على الثقة والاحترام المتبادل ، فإن توجيه أصابع الاتهام عندما لا تعرف على وجه اليقين لا يؤدي إلا إلى خلق دراما غير ضرورية ، لذا تحقق بدقة .عندما يكون لديك حقائقك على التوالي ، يمكنك مناقشة كل ما قد تكون اكتشفته بهدوء.

Avoid Unneeded Chaos

Evite el caos innecesario

تجنب الفوضى غير الضرورية

We tend to hurt the ones we love. We take out anger from work, and it trickles down to others. When we are mindful of our tendency to do things like this, we can break the habit.

While we want to share our feelings and emotions, maybe we hold the drama for a few. Say hello first, give each other a kiss or something nice before launching into the daily drama. Don't let your drama bring down others if you can avoid it, so be selective in sharing drama.

Even though it may be something we want to vent off our chest, will our venting negatively impact others around us? If the answer is yes, ask yourself how necessary it is to create drama. If drama can be avoided, then focus on the positive and finding solutions.

Tendemos a lastimar a los que amamos. Sacamos la ira del trabajo y se filtra a los demás. Cuando somos conscientes de nuestra tendencia a hacer cosas como esta, podemos romper el hábito.

Si bien queremos compartir nuestros sentimientos y emociones, tal vez mantengamos el drama por unos pocos. Saludaos primero, dáganse un beso o algo agradable antes de lanzarse al drama diario. No dejes que tu drama derribe a otros si puedes evitarlo, así que sé selectivo al compartir el drama.

A pesar de que puede ser algo que queremos desahogar de nuestro pecho, ¿nuestro desahogo afectará negativamente a los que nos rodean? Si la respuesta es sí, pregúntate qué tan necesario es crear drama. Si se puede evitar el drama, concéntrese en lo positivo y encuentre soluciones.

نحن نميل إلى إيذاء من نحبهم. نحن نخرج الغضب من العمل ، ويتدفق إلى الآخرين. عندما نضع في اعتبارنا ميلنا للقيام بأشياء كهذه، يمكننا كسر هذه العادة.

بينما نريد مشاركة مشاعرنا وعواطفنا ، ربما نحتفظ بالدراما لعدد قليل. قل مرحبا أولا ، وأعط بعضنا البعض قبلة أو شيئا لطيفا قبل الانطلاق في الدراما اليومية. لا تدع الدراما الخاصة بك تسقط الآخرين إذا كنت تستطيع تجنبها ، لذا كن انتقائيا في مشاركة الدراما.

على الرغم من أنه قد يكون شيئا نريد التنفيس عنه من صدرنا فهل سيؤثر تنفيسنا سلبا على الآخرين من حولنا؟ إذا كانت الإجابة بنعم ، اسأل نفسك عن مدى ضرورة إنشاء دراما. إذا

كان من الممكن تجنب الدراما ، فركز على الحلول الإيجابية
وإيجاد الحلول.

Let Them Overshare

Déjelos compartir en exceso

دعهم يبالغون في المشاركة

If you lover wants to vent or tell a long-winded story, let them say it. Don't roll your eyes, huff, sigh, or tell them to be quiet. You never know when you might want to vent, too.

That's the give and take of a relationship. Sometimes, people need to vent. Let it out.

Taking the time to listen increases the bond. Shared experiences, such as dates, creating memories are the little things that strengthen a bond that makes sex that much more amazing. Beyond the mere function of in and out, there's the emotions that are created over time as well.

Si tu amante quiere desahogarse o contar una historia de largo aliento, deja que lo diga. No pongas los ojos en blanco, resoplés, suspires ni les digas que se callen. *Nunca se sabe cuándo es posible que desee desahogarse, también.*

Ese es el toma y daca de una relación. A veces, las personas necesitan desahogarse. Déjalo salir.

Tomarse el tiempo para escuchar aumenta el vínculo. Las experiencias compartidas, como las citas, la creación de recuerdos son las pequeñas cosas que fortalecen un vínculo que hace que el sexo sea mucho más increíble. Más allá de la mera función de entrar y salir, también están las emociones que se crean con el tiempo.

إذا كنت تحب التنفيس أو رواية قصة طويلة ، فدعه يقول ذلك. لا تدحرج عينيك أو تتنهد أو تتنهد أو تطلب منهما أن يكونا هادئين. أنت لا تعرف أبدا متى قد ترغب في التنفيس أيضا.

هذا هو الأخذ والعطاء للعلاقة. في بعض الأحيان ، يحتاج الناس إلى التنفيس. دعها تخرج.

أخذ الوقت الكافي للاستماع يزيد من الرابطة. التجارب المشتركة ، مثل التواريخ ، وخلق الذكريات هي الأشياء الصغيرة التي تقوي الرابطة التي تجعل الجنس أكثر إثارة للدهشة. بالإضافة إلى مجرد وظيفة الدخول والخروج ، هناك العواطف التي يتم إنشاؤها بمرور الوقت أيضا.

Turn Off Frequencies

Desactivar frecuencias

إيقاف تشغيل الترددات

Taking the time to really listen includes turning off the frequencies to provide your full attention. It's hard to bond when someone has their face buried in their phone or computer. Turn off the electronics for a moment, and really take the time to make eye contact with each other, as the eyes are the first point of attraction, when you make eye contact and realize.

Eye contact, facial expressions and body language can break language barriers. Someone does not have to speak the same language to understand when someone is interested. It's a matter of approaching the situation correctly, not being too overly aggressive excited.

Pursed lips, raised eyebrows, blushing smiles, head nods and more are telltale signs. When a person is staring at a screen, they miss those subtle body motions and language. Twirling hair, giggling, locking eyes without looking away, and biting lips may be seen.

Tomarse el tiempo para escuchar realmente incluye apagar las frecuencias para proporcionar toda su atención. Es difícil vincularse cuando alguien tiene la cara enterrada en su teléfono o computadora. Apague la electrónica por un momento, y realmente tómese el tiempo para hacer contacto visual entre sí, ya que los ojos son el primer punto de atracción, cuando hace contacto visual y se da cuenta.

El contacto visual, las expresiones faciales y el lenguaje corporal pueden romper las barreras del idioma. Alguien no tiene que hablar el mismo idioma para entender cuando alguien está interesado. Es cuestión de abordar la situación correctamente, no ser demasiado agresivo emocionado.

Labios fruncidos, cejas arqueadas, sonrisas sonrojadas, asentimientos con la cabeza y más son signos reveladores. Cuando una persona está mirando una pantalla, se pierde esos movimientos corporales sutiles y el lenguaje. Se puede ver el cabello girando, riendo, cerrando los ojos sin mirar hacia otro lado y mordiéndose los labios.

يتضمن أخذ الوقت الكافي للاستماع حقا إيقاف تشغيل الترددات لتوفير انتباهك الكامل. من الصعب الارتباط عندما يكون شخص ما قد دفن وجهه في هاتفه أو جهاز الكمبيوتر الخاص به. قم بايقاف تشغيل الإلكترونيات للحظة وخذ الوقت الكافي لإجراء اتصال بصري مع بعضها ،

البعض ، لأن العينين هما نقطة الجذب الأولى ، عندما تقوم بالاتصال البصري وتدرك.

يمكن أن يؤدي الاتصال البصري وتعبيرات الوجه ولغة الجسد إلى كسر الحواجز اللغوية. لا يتعين على شخص ما التحدث بنفس اللغة لفهم متى يكون شخص ما مهتما. إنها مسألة الاقتراب من الموقف بشكل صحيح ، وليس الإثارة العدوانية المفرطة.

الشفاه المسحوبة ، والحواجب المرفوعة ، والابتسامات الحمرة ، وإيماءات الرأس وأكثر من ذلك هي علامات منبهة. عندما يحدق شخص ما في الشاشة ، فإنه يفتقد حركات الجسم الدقيقة واللغة. يمكن رؤية الشعر الدوار ، والضحك ، وقفل العينين دون النظر بعيدا ، والشفاه العض.

One and Only

Uno y único

واحد وفقط

Make you lover feel as if they are your one and only, even if they are not — especially if they are not. Do not ask your lover for condoms or talk about other lovers. Do not compare them to other past or present lovers.

Do not look at other lovers on your phone or have shady conversations behind your lover's back.

Instead, act as if they mean the world to you, as that makes them feel good, and the good feelings will trickle down the bedroom. However, there is a saying, "hell has no fury like a scorned woman," so don't test that theory at all.

Mentioning and implying others only builds jealousy and resentment. It starts the one-upsman game, of if you than do that, then I can do even better than you, starting the spiteful battle of tit for tat. Instead of opening that Pandora's Box, just make them feel special.

Haz que tu amante se sienta como si fuera tu único y único, incluso si no lo son, especialmente si no lo son. No le pidas condones a tu amante ni hables de otros amantes. No los compares con otros amantes pasados o presentes.

No mires a otros amantes en tu teléfono ni tengas conversaciones turbias a espaldas de tu amante. En su lugar, actúe como si significaran el mundo para usted, ya que eso los hace sentir bien, y los buenos sentimientos se filtrarán por el dormitorio. Sin embargo, hay un dicho, "el infierno no tiene furia como una mujer despreciada", así que no pruebes esa teoría en absoluto.

Mencionar e implicar a otros solo genera celos y resentimiento. Comienza el juego de un solo hombre, de si haces eso, entonces puedo hacerlo

incluso mejor que tú, comenzando la batalla
rencorosa de teta por teta. En lugar de abrir esa caja
de Pandora, solo haz que se sientan especiales.

، اجعلك حبيبا يشعر كما لو كان هو الوحيد والوحيد
حتى لو لم يكن كذلك ـ خاصة إذا لم يكن كذلك .لا تسأل
حبيبك عن الواقي الذكري أو تتحدث عن عشاق آخرين .لا
.تقارنهم بعشاق الماضي أو الحاضر الآخرين

لا تنظر إلى العشاق الآخرين على هاتفك أو تجري
محادثات مشبوهة خلف ظهر حبيبك .بدلا من ذلك ، تصرف
كما لو أنهم يعنون العالم بالنسبة لك ، لأن ذلك يجعلهم
يشعرون بالرضا ، وسوف تتسرب المشاعر الجيدة إلى
غرفة النوم .ومع ذلك ، هناك قول مأثور ،"الجحيم ليس لديه
غضب مثل امرأة محتقرة"، لذلك لا تختبر هذه النظرية على
.الإطلاق

إن ذكر الآخرين والإيحاء بهم لا يؤدي إلا إلى بناء
الغيرة والاستياء .إنها تبدأ لعبة الوداع الواحد ، إذا كنت
تفعل ذلك ، فيمكنني أن أفعل أفضل منك ، وأبدأ المعركة
الحاقدة من الحلمة من أجل التات .بدلا من فتح صندوق
.باندورا، فقط اجعلهم يشعرون بأنهم مميزون

In The Bedroom

En el dormitorio

في غرفة النوم

Creating A Spark

Creación de una chispa

خلق شرارة

A gentle touch can create interest, especially when in a non-sexual place, such as a slight brush on the forearm, a brief pat on the shoulder, or a brief finger along their hand. The point is not to mount someone or slam it in as fast as possible. The point is to create interest.

Human contact trumps electronic interaction. Touch is a sensation to be tantalized. Tease, take your time with it, like hunting a prey, slowly taking your time before pouncing.

Do not rush it. Draw it out. Make them want you more.

Un toque suave puede crear interés, especialmente cuando se encuentra en un lugar no sexual, como un ligero cepillo en el antebrazo, una breve palmadita en el hombro o un breve dedo a lo largo de la mano. El punto no es montar a alguien o golpearlo lo más rápido posible. El punto es crear interés.

El contacto humano triunfa sobre la interacción electrónica. El tacto es una sensación para ser tentado. Burlarse, tómese su tiempo con él, como cazar una presa, tomarse lentamente su tiempo antes de saltar.

No te apresures. Sácalo. Haz que te quieran más.

يمكن أن تخلق اللمسة اللطيفة اهتماما ، خاصة عندما تكون في مكان غير جنسي ، مثل فرشاة طفيفة على الساعد ، أو ربت قصير على الكتف ، أو إصبع قصير على طول يده. الهدف ليس تركيب شخص ما أو ضربه في أسرع وقت ممكن. الهدف هو خلق الاهتمام.

الاتصال البشري يتفوق على التفاعل الإلكتروني. اللمس هو إحساس يجب تحريكه. ندف ، خذ وقتك معها ، مثل صيد فريسة ، خذ وقتك ببطء قبل الصيد.

لا تتعجل ذلك. اسحبها. اجعلهم يريدونك أكثر.

Kiss Body Parts

Besar partes del cuerpo

قبلة أجزاء الجسم

Once you have secured a spot heading towards the bedroom, you can kick up the contact to kissing. While French kissing is always amazing, be sure to kiss other body parts as well. Massaging and kissing intimately would be what is called foreplay.

It's like warming up the engine. Taking a few minutes ahead of time will make the whole thing run smoother over time. Tantalize random body parts.

Kiss the back of the neck, nibble on the ear lobes, with a slightly intentional small breath in their ear, so they can feel the warm, moist breath make hairs rise. Gently dragging nails along the skin, barely touching in such a manner that makes them squirm with delight, kiss just as delicately. Tease and build up their desire.

Una vez que haya asegurado un lugar que se dirija hacia el dormitorio, puede levantar el contacto para besarse. Si bien los besos franceses siempre son increíbles, asegúrese de besar otras partes del cuerpo también. Masajear y besarse íntimamente sería lo que se llama juego previo.

Es como calentar el motor. Tomar unos minutos antes de tiempo hará que todo funcione más suavemente con el tiempo. Tentar partes aleatorias del cuerpo.

Bese la parte posterior del cuello, mordisquee los lóbulos de las orejas, con una pequeña respiración ligeramente intencional en su oído, para que puedan sentir que el aliento cálido y húmedo hace que los pelos se levanten. Arrastrando suavemente las uñas a lo largo de la piel, apenas tocándolas de tal manera que las haga retorcerse de deleite, besar con la misma delicadeza. Burlarse y construir su deseo.

بمجرد تأمين مكان متجه نحو غرفة النوم ، يمكنك تحريك جهة الاتصال إلى التقبيل. في حين أن التقبيل الفرنسي دائما ما يكون مذهلا ، تأكد من تقبيل أجزاء الجسم الأخرى أيضا. سيكون التدليك والتقبيل بشكل حميم ما يسمى المداعبة.

انها مثل تسخين المحرك. إن أخذ بضع دقائق في وقت مبكر سيجعل الأمر برمته أكثر سلاسة بمرور الوقت. تحمير أجزاء الجسم العشوائية.

تقبيل الجزء الخلفي من الرقبة ، قضم على فصوص الأذن مع نفس صغير متعمد قليلا في أذنهم ، حتى يتمكنوا من الشعور بالتنفس الدافئ والرطب يجعل الشعر يرتفع. سحب الأظافر بلطف على طول الجلد ، بالكاد لمس بطريقة تجعلها تتلوى بسرور ، وتقبيل بنفس القدر من الدقة. مضايقة وبناء رغبتهم.

Nibble Ear Lobes

Mordisquear los lóbulos de la oreja

قضم فصوص الأذن

Don't chomp and bite, but a gentle pressure of the teeth on the earlobe, followed by a puff of hot breath, may be just enough to send shivers of excitement. It's not like you have to tongue out their ears, as it's not about cleaning the wax out or slobbering in their ears. Think of it as a playful taunt, a barely there feeling.

Following up with gentle kisses on the neck, even gently caressing the hair and face. Again, it's not about licking them clean. It's a subtle stimulation, almost tickling, the barely there is what can make the hair rise.

Gently massaging the ears does not digging inside for buried treasure, but stimulating the outside of the earlobe. Barely touch around the outside of the ear, from top to bottom, then follow that up with oral stimulation. Hands move to the hair, as the tongue meets the ear lobe, teeth barely scraping the skin.

No muerda y muerda, pero una presión suave de los dientes en el lóbulo de la oreja, seguida de una bocanada de aliento caliente, puede ser suficiente para enviar escalofríos de emoción. No es como si tuvieras que sacarles las orejas, ya que no se trata de limpiar la cera o babear en sus oídos. Piense en ello como una burla juguetona, un sentimiento que apenas existe.

Siguiendo con besos suaves en el cuello, incluso acariciando suavemente el cabello y la cara. Una vez más, no se trata de lamerlos limpios. Es una estimulación sutil, casi cosquilleante, lo que apenas hay es lo que puede hacer que el cabello se eleve.

Masajear suavemente las orejas no cava dentro en busca de tesoros enterrados, sino estimular el exterior del lóbulo de la oreja. Apenas toque alrededor del exterior del oído, de arriba a abajo, luego siga con estimulación oral. Las manos se mueven hacia el cabello, a medida que la lengua se encuentra con el lóbulo de la oreja, los dientes apenas raspan la piel.

لا تخنق وتعض ، ولكن الضغط اللطيف للأسنان على شحمة الأذن ، متبوعا بنفخة من التنفس الساخن ، قد يكون كافيا لإرسال ارتعاشات من الإثارة . ليس الأمر كما لو كان عليك أن تخرج آذانهم ، لأن الأمر لا يتعلق بتنظيف الشمع أو

، اللطخة في آذانهم .فكر في الأمر على أنه سخرية مرحة
.شعور بالكاد هناك

المتابعة مع قبلات لطيفة على الرقبة ، حتى مداعبة
الشعر والوجه بلطف .مرة أخرى ، لا يتعلق الأمر بلعقها
نظيفة .إنه تحفيز دقيق ، يكاد يكون دغدغة ، بالكاد يوجد ما
.يمكن أن يجعل الشعر يرتفع

تدليك الأذنين بلطف لا يحفر في الداخل بحثا عن كنز مدفون
ولكن يحفز الجزء الخارجي من شحمة الأذن .بالكاد تلمس ،
حول الجزء الخارجي من الأذن ، من أعلى إلى أسفل ، ثم
اتبع ذلك بالتحفيز الفموي .تتحرك الأيدي إلى الشعر ، حيث
.يلتقي اللسان بشحمة الأذن ، والأسنان بالكاد تكشط الجلد

Stimulate Unexpected Areas

Estimular áreas inesperadas

تحفيز المناطق غير المتوقعة

A gentle stimulation on the inside of the
elbow or the back of the knee, such as kiss or nails
barely dragged across the skin, is an example of an
unexpected area. Definitely kiss the lips, as well as
the inner thigh. The feet can be a playground of
stimulation for those brave.

Find areas normally ignored, such as the
underside of breasts where underwire bra straps rub

raw. Suck there for a few moments to surprise with sensation. There's also the crevasse where underwear rubs.

Head, face and neck massages, very gently, can be stimulating, as well as relieving if a partner has migraines. Rubbing the temples and jawline can be soothing. Always start with gentle sensations.

Una estimulación suave en el interior del codo o la parte posterior de la rodilla, como un beso o uñas apenas arrastradas por la piel, es un ejemplo de un área inesperada. Definitivamente besa los labios, así como la parte interna del muslo. Los pies pueden ser un patio de recreo de estimulación para aquellos valientes.

Encuentre áreas normalmente ignoradas, como la parte inferior de los senos donde las correas del sostén con alambre se frotan crudas. Chupa allí por unos momentos para sorprender con sensación. También está la grieta donde se frota la ropa interior.

Los masajes de cabeza, cara y cuello, muy suavemente, pueden ser estimulantes, además de aliviar si una pareja tiene migrañas. Frotar las sienes y la mandíbula puede ser calmante. Comience siempre con sensaciones suaves.

، التحفيز اللطيف داخل الكوع أو الجزء الخلفي من الركبة مثل القبلة أو الأظافر التي بالكاد يتم سحبها عبر الجلد ، هو مثال على منطقة غير متوقعة. بالتأكيد تقبيل الشفاه ، وكذلك الفخذ الداخلي. يمكن أن تكون القدمين ملعبا للتحفيز لأولئك الشجعان.

ابحثي عن المناطق التي يتم تجاهلها عادة، مثل الجانب السفلي من الثديين حيث تفرك أحزمة حمالة الصدر السفلية نيئة. تمتص هناك لبضع لحظات لتفاجئ بالإحساس. هناك أيضا الصدع حيث تحتك الملابس الداخلية.

يمكن أن يكون تدليك الرأس والوجه والرقبة ، بلطف شديد محفزا ، وكذلك يخفف إذا كان الشريك يعاني من الصداع النصفي. فرك المعابد وخط الفك يمكن أن يكون مهدئا. ابدأ دائما بأحاسيس لطيفة.

Best French Kisses

Los mejores besos franceses

أفضل القبلات الفرنسية

French kisses are when the tongues of two individuals are intertwined. Try not to be overly sloppy like a drooling dog, but rub tongues with a gentle suck. Don't be too gentle like you are kissing your grandmother, but don't be too aggressive like you're trying to suck your partner's face off either.

Try not to knock teeth, as that creates a nails-on-chalkboard sensation that is not always fun. Instead, you can try rubbing your tongue on your partner's teeth. Have fun with French kissing, and explore the orifice.

Rub your tongue on the roof of your partner's mouth. Suck their bottom lip. Stare into their eyes.

Los besos franceses son cuando las lenguas de dos individuos están entrelazadas. Trate de no ser demasiado descuidado como un perro babeante, pero frote las lenguas con una succión suave. No seas demasiado gentil como si estuvieras besando a tu abuela, pero tampoco seas demasiado agresivo como si estuvieras tratando de chupar la cara de tu pareja.

Trate de no golpear los dientes, ya que eso crea una sensación de uñas en la pizarra que no siempre es divertida. En su lugar, puede intentar frotar su lengua en los dientes de su pareja. Diviértete con besos franceses y explora el orificio.

Frote la lengua en el techo de la boca de su pareja. Chupa su labio inferior. Mirarlos a los ojos.

القبلات الفرنسية هي عندما تتشابك ألسنة شخصين. حاول ألا تكون قذرا بشكل مفرط مثل يسيل لعابه ، ولكن افرك

الألسنة بمص لطيف .لا تكن لطيفا جدا كما لو كنت تقبل جدتك ، ولكن لا تكن عدوانيا جدا كما لو كنت تحاول امتصاص وجه شريكك أيضا.

حاول ألا تدق الأسنان ، لأن ذلك يخلق إحساسا بالأظافر على السبورة ليس ممتعا دائما .بدلا من ذلك ، يمكنك محاولة فرك لسانك على أسنان شريكك .استمتع بالتقبيل الفرنسي واستكشف الفتحة.

افرك لسانك على سطح فم شريكك .مص شفتهم السفلية .يحدقون في أعينهم.

Flicking the Bean

Moviendo el frijol

نفض الغبار عن الفول

When pleasing a woman, stimulating the clitoris is very important, especially if you're trying to enter the back door, always keep that stimulated, just another tip. Many people have problems finding the clit, as it is hidden under folds of labia skin and is about the size of a bean. Some people refer to it as the man in the boat, as if you're looking at a vagina as being like a row boat, towards the top, where the flaps and folds of skin start, that is like the top of the canoe, and up there, if you peel back the waves of skin, you will reveal that bean-sized clit that juts out like a man in a boat would sitting up.

With lubrication, rubbing that in a circular motion is great stimulation, but if doing oral, you want to flick that bean with your tongue, back and forth lightly, and it's almost like the lighter you touch it, the more intense it gets, as if being tickled. Thus, if using a dildo for stimulation, while many might grind when it gets good, to really start stimulation, do not press hard at all, but lightly touch the vibrating object to the clit. Just barely touch it, and you should get a reaction, especially if it is fully exposed, skin flaps folded back.

Sucking on the clit as if you are ravenously hungry can be another effective maneuver, but be careful not to bite hard or draw blood, as the area is sensitive. People suggest drawing the alphabet with your tongue on the clit as a way to start oral sex, while others might add lubrication and a vibrator; still, there's an entire segment of the population that doesn't do oral sex. Individual preferences vary, and they can vary at convenient times as well, but when in doubt, ask, though people will generally tell you if they do not want it.

Al complacer a una mujer, estimular el clítoris es muy importante, especialmente si estás tratando de entrar por la puerta trasera, siempre mantén eso estimulado, solo otro consejo. Muchas personas tienen problemas para encontrar el clítoris, ya que está oculto debajo de los pliegues de la piel de los labios y es aproximadamente del tamaño de un frijol. Algunas personas se refieren a él como el hombre en el bote, como si estuvieras mirando una vagina como si fuera un bote de remos, hacia la parte superior, donde comienzan las solapas y los pliegues de la piel, es decir, la parte superior de la canoa, y allí arriba, si pelas las olas de piel, revelarás ese clítoris del tamaño de un frijol que sobresale como lo haría un hombre en un bote.

Con la lubricación, frotar eso en un movimiento circular es una gran estimulación, pero si lo haces por vía oral, quieres mover ese frijol con la lengua, de un lado a otro ligeramente, y es casi como cuanto más ligero lo tocas, más intenso se vuelve, como si te hicieran cosquillas. Por lo tanto, si usa un consolador para la estimulación, aunque muchos pueden moler cuando se pone bueno, para realmente comenzar la estimulación, no presione con fuerza en absoluto, sino que toque ligeramente el objeto vibratorio al clítoris.

Apenas lo toca, y debería obtener una reacción, especialmente si está completamente expuesto, las solapas de la piel dobladas hacia atrás.

Chupar el clítoris como si tuvieras hambre voraz puede ser otra maniobra efectiva, pero ten cuidado de no morder con fuerza o extraer sangre, ya que el área es sensible. La gente sugiere dibujar el

alfabeto con la lengua en el clítoris como una forma
de comenzar el sexo oral, mientras que otros pueden
agregar lubricación y un vibrador; aún así, hay todo
un segmento de la población que no hace sexo oral.
Las preferencias individuales varían, y también
pueden variar en momentos convenientes, pero en
caso de duda, pregunte, aunque las personas
generalmente le dirán si no lo quieren.

عند إرضاء المرأة ، فإن تحفيز البظر مهم جدا ، خاصة إذا
كنت تحاول دخول الباب الخلفي ، فحافظ دائما على تحفيز
ذلك ، مجرد نصيحة أخرى. كثير من الناس لديهم مشاكل في
العثور على البظر ، لأنه مخفي تحت طيات جلد الشفرين
ويبلغ حجمه حوالي حجم الفول. يشير بعض الناس إليه على
أنه الرجل في القارب ، كما لو كنت تنظر إلى المهبل على أنه
مثل قارب التجديف ، نحو الأعلى ، حيث تبدأ اللوحات
، والطيات الجلدية ، وهذا يشبه الجزء العلوي من الزورق
وإلى هناك ، إذا قمت بتقشير موجات الجلد ، فسوف تكشف
عن البظر بحجم الفاصوليا الذي يبرز مثل رجل في قارب
يجلس.

، مع التشحيم ، يعد فرك ذلك في حركة دائرية تحفيزا رائعا
ولكن إذا كنت تفعل عن طريق الفم ، فأنت تريد أن تنقر تلك
الفولة بلسانك ، ذهابا وإيابا بخفة ، وهي تشبه تقريبا كلما
لمستها أخف وزنا ، كلما زادت كثافتها ، كما لو كانت
مدغدغة. وبالتالي ، إذا كنت تستخدم دسارا للتحفيز ، في
حين أن الكثيرين قد يطحنون عندما يصبح جيدا ، لبدء
التحفيز حقا ، لا تضغط بقوة على الإطلاق ، ولكن المس
الكائن المهتز برفق إلى البظر.

بالكاد تلمسه ، ويجب أن تحصل على رد فعل ، خاصة إذا كان مكشوفا بالكامل ، ولوحات الجلد مطوية للخلف.

يمكن أن يكون مص البظر كما لو كنت جائعا بشدة مناورة فعالة أخرى ، ولكن احرص على عدم العض بقوة أو سحب الدم ، لأن المنطقة حساسة .يقترح الناس رسم الأبجدية مع لسانك على البظر كوسيلة لبدء ممارسة الجنس عن طريق الفم ، في حين أن الآخرين قد يضيفون التشحيم والهزاز .ومع ذلك ، هناك شريحة كاملة من السكان لا تمارس الجنس عن طريق الفم .تختلف التفضيلات الفردية ، ويمكن أن تختلف في أوقات مناسبة أيضا ، ولكن عندما تكون في شك ، اسأل على الرغم من أن الناس سيخبرونك عموما إذا كانوا لا يريدون ذلك.

That Space Underneath

Ese espacio debajo

تلك المساحة تحتها

With guys, there's that space underneath the ball sack, just before the anus, that can be stimulated. Rubbing in a circular motion with the thumb while giving oral stimulation, or even sucking up and stimulating with the tongue if tossing the salad, can be pleasurable. Cuff the balls, lightly stimulate the nuts.

The head of the penis can be the most sensitive. Light flickers of the tongue here can be a great start. Tease a little, before swallowing the whole cock at once.

Light and loose, or fast and hard sucking, the preference can vary from person to person. Thus, there's no universal way to be able to do it right. Some like teeth, feeling as if they will be swallowed up, while others prefer the light as a feather, or slow and steady.

Con los chicos, hay ese espacio debajo del saco de pelota, justo antes del ano, que se puede estimular. Frotar en un movimiento circular con el pulgar mientras se da estimulación oral, o incluso succionar y estimular con la lengua si se lanza la ensalada, puede ser placentero. Tape las bolas, estimule ligeramente las nueces.

La cabeza del pene puede ser la más sensible. Los ligeros parpadeos de la lengua aquí pueden ser un gran comienzo. Burlarse un poco, antes de tragar toda la polla a la vez.

Ligera y suelta, o succión rápida y dura, la preferencia puede variar de persona a persona. Por lo tanto, no hay una forma universal de poder hacerlo bien. A algunos les gustan los dientes, sintiendo como si fueran tragados, mientras que

otros prefieren la luz como una pluma, o lenta y
constante.

مع الرجال ، هناك تلك المساحة تحت كيس الكرة ، قبل فتحة الشرج مباشرة ، والتي يمكن تحفيزها. فرك في حركة دائرية مع الإبهام أثناء إعطاء التحفيز عن طريق الفم ، أو حتى مص وتحفيز مع اللسان إذا رمي السلطة ، يمكن أن يكون ممتعا. الكفة الكرات ، وتحفيز المكسرات بخفة.

يمكن أن يكون رأس القضيب هو الأكثر حساسية. يمكن أن تكون الوميض الخفيف للسان هنا بداية رائعة. ندف قليلا ، قبل ابتلاع الديك كله في وقت واحد.

خفيف وفضفاض ، أو مص سريع وصعب ، يمكن أن يختلف التفضيل من شخص لآخر. وبالتالي ، لا توجد طريقة عالمية لتكون قادرا على القيام بذلك بشكل صحيح. يحب البعض الأسنان ، ويشعرون كما لو أنهم سيتم ابتلاعها ، بينما يفضل آخرون الضوء كريشة ، أو بطيء وثابت.

The Kinky Stuff

Las cosas pervertidas

الاثياء الغريبة

On Sexual Strangulation
Sobre el estrangulamiento sexual
حول الخنق الجنسي

Some of you are thinking that sexual strangulation is something fun to try, but you have to realize the dangers that are involved in it. First off, you must be mindful of the windpipe and esophagus. Trying this technique the wrong way can definitely damage those things permanently, and if you hold on too long, you can literally kill someone when doing it.

Take it from the girl, me, who had to have CPR done on her to bring her back to life after a guy held on a little too long. He was intoxicated, thinking about his own pleasure, and next thing you know, I was not moving or breathing, so he had to do CPR to revive me. That moment of panic during sex is a warning to all.

That being said, if you are still going to do it, at least do the two-handed technique, palms on either side of the windpipe, careful not to crush it, palms facing out. If you insist on trying one-handed, at least cup upward to not crush the windpipe, merely pinching the jugular closed on

either side, as that's what is happening during
sexual strangulation, you cut off blood supply to the
brain, as well as air supply, causing you to pass out.

Algunos de ustedes están pensando que el
estrangulamiento sexual es algo divertido de probar,
pero tienen que darse cuenta de los peligros que están
involucrados en ello. En primer lugar, debe tener en
cuenta la tráquea y el esófago. Probar esta técnica
de la manera incorrecta definitivamente puede dañar
esas cosas permanentemente, y si te aferras
demasiado tiempo, literalmente puedes matar a
alguien cuando lo haces.

Tómelo de la chica, yo, que tuvo que hacerse
RCP para devolverla a la vida después de que un
chico aguantó demasiado tiempo. Estaba
intoxicado, pensando en su propio placer, y lo
siguiente que sabes, no me movía ni respiraba, así
que tuvo que hacer RCP para revivirme. Ese
momento de pánico durante el sexo es una
advertencia para todos.

Dicho esto, si todavía lo vas a hacer, al
menos haz la técnica a dos manos, palmas a cada
lado de la tráquea, cuidado de no aplastarla, palmas
hacia afuera. Si insistes en intentar con una sola
mano, al menos una taza hacia arriba para no
aplastar la tráquea, simplemente pellizcando la
yugular cerrada a ambos lados, ya que eso es lo que
está sucediendo durante el estrangulamiento sexual,

cortas el suministro de sangre al cerebro, así como el
suministro de aire, lo que hace que te desmayes.

يعتقد بعضكم أن الخنق الجنسي شيء ممتع لتجربته ، ولكن
عليك أن تدرك المخاطر التي تنطوي عليه .أولا ، يجب أن
تضع في اعتبارك القصبة الهوائية والمريء .إن تجربة هذه
التقنية بطريقة خاطئة يمكن أن تلحق الضرر بهذه الأشياء
بشكل دائم ، وإذا صمدت لفترة طويلة جدا ، فيمكنك حرفيا
قتل شخص ما عند القيام بذلك.

خذها من الفتاة ، أنا ، التي اضطرت إلى إجراء الإنعاش
القلبي الرئوي عليها لإعادتها إلى الحياة بعد أن تمسك بها
رجل لفترة طويلة جدا .كان مخمورا ، يفكر في متعته
الخاصة ، والشيء التالي الذي تعرفه ، لم أكن أتحرك أو
أتنفس ، لذلك كان عليه أن يفعل الإنعاش القلبي الرئوي
لإحيائي .لحظة الذعر هذه أثناء ممارسة الجنس هي تحذير
للجميع.

ومع ذلك ، إذا كنت لا تزال ستفعل ذلك ، على الأقل قم بتقنية
اليدين ، والنخيل على جانبي القصبة الهوائية ، والحرص
على عدم سحقها ، والنخيل تواجه الخارج .إذا كنت تصر
على محاولة بيد واحدة ، على الأقل كوب لأعلى لعدم سحق
القصبة الهوائية ، مجرد قرص الوداجي مغلق على كلا
الجانبين ، لأن هذا ما يحدث أثناء الخنق الجنسي ، فإنك تقطع
إمدادات الدم إلى الدماغ ، وكذلك إمدادات الهواء ، مما يسبب
لك الإغماء.

Slave and Master

Esclavo y Amo

العبد والسيد

Do not pretend to be into bondage if you are not, as you might not like the surprises you get in the bedroom if you do not realize what it entails. A submissive is called a slave, and a dominant is called a master. Some people like to play both roles, and they are called switch.

Switch also refers to being bisexual in some communities, and in the gay male community, a switch is someone who will be either a bottom or a top in sex. The bottom is typically the female role, the receiver, while the top is more of the stereotypical male role, the penis giver. The bottom is called the female role as they are the ones that are being penetrated in their mangina or asshole.

In bondage, the master typically will dominate the slave, which may include whips, being chained up, having ice cubes rubbed on the skin, followed by hot candle wax, and even electronic shock through piercings. The goal is the discover the line between pleasure and pain, as well as learning your own personal boundaries.

No finjas estar en esclavitud si no lo estás, ya que es posible que no te gusten las sorpresas que recibes en el dormitorio si no te das cuenta de lo que implica. Un sumiso se llama esclavo, y un dominante se llama amo. A algunas personas les gusta desempeñar ambos roles, y se les llama interruptor.

Switch también se refiere a ser bisexual en algunas comunidades, y en la comunidad masculina gay, un switch es alguien que será un inferior o un superior en el sexo. La parte inferior es típicamente el papel femenino, el receptor, mientras que la parte superior es más del papel masculino estereotipado, el dador del pene. La parte inferior se llama el papel femenino ya que son las que están siendo penetradas en su mangina o gilipollas.

En la esclavitud, el amo generalmente dominará al esclavo, lo que puede incluir látigos, estar encadenado, frotar cubitos de hielo en la piel, seguido de cera de vela caliente e incluso choque electrónico a través de perforaciones. El objetivo es descubrir la línea entre el placer y el dolor, así como aprender sus propios límites personales.

لا تتظاهر بأنك في عبودية إذا لم تكن كذلك ، لأنك قد لا تحب المفاجآت التي تحصل عليها في غرفة النوم إذا لم تدرك ما ينطوي عليه. يسمى الخاضع عبدا ، ويسمى المهيمن سيدا.

بعض الناس يحبون أن يلعبوا كلا الدورين ، ويطلق عليهم التبديل.

يشير Switch أيضا إلى كونك ثنائي الجنس في بعض المجتمعات ، وفي مجتمع الذكور المثليين ، فإن التبديل هو شخص سيكون إما في القاع أو القمة في الجنس. الجزء السفلي هو عادة دور الأنثى ، المتلقي ، في حين أن الجزء العلوي هو أكثر من دور الذكور النمطي ، مانح القضيب. يسمى الجزء السفلي دور الأنثى لأنها هي التي يتم اختراقها في المانجينا أو الأحمق.

في العبودية ، عادة ما يهيمن السيد على العبد ، والذي قد يشمل السياط ، والسلاسل ، وفرك مكعبات الثلج على الجلد تليها شمع الشموع الساخن ، وحتى الصدمة الإلكترونية من خلال الثقوب. الهدف هو اكتشاف الخط الفاصل بين المتعة والألم ، وكذلك تعلم حدودك الشخصية.

Get Blind-Folded

Ponte los ojos vendados

الحصول على معصوب العينين

When people think of bondage, many think of being tied up and blindfolded. There are many break-away handcuffs that mimic the sensation of being tied up, but if someone starts to panic, they can break away. The concept of being blind-folded does not have to include being tied up, but they go hand in hand mostly.

The point of being tied up is to allow your partner to have complete control of your body, and you have enough trust in your partner to know you will not be harmed. It's a complete surrender. Take me now.

Do whatever you want with me, penetrate any hole in any way, or don't penetrate at all, that's the suspense of being blind-folded and tied up is that you don't know what is going to happen, and you cannot resist it from happening either. If someone cuffs you to a spinning rack and wants to spin you until you puke, they can. They might just surprise you with whips and ice, and that's the nature of the beast, not knowing what your partner will do, and waiting with anticipation.

Cuando la gente piensa en la esclavitud, muchos piensan en estar atados y con los ojos vendados. Hay muchas esposas que imitan la sensación de estar atado, pero si alguien comienza a entrar en pánico, puede romper. El concepto de tener los ojos vendados no tiene por qué incluir estar atado, pero van de la mano en su mayoría.

El objetivo de estar atado es permitir que su pareja tenga un control completo de su cuerpo, y usted tiene suficiente confianza en su pareja para saber que no será perjudicado. Es una rendición completa. Llévame ahora.

Haz lo que quieras conmigo, penetra en cualquier agujero de cualquier manera, o no penetres en absoluto, ese es el suspenso de estar con los ojos vendados y atados es que no sabes lo que va a suceder, y tampoco puedes resistirte a que suceda. Si alguien te esposa a un estante giratorio y quiere girarte hasta que vomites, puede hacerlo. Es posible que simplemente te sorprendan con látigos y hielo, y esa es la naturaleza de la bestia, sin saber lo que hará tu pareja y esperando con anticipación.

عندما يفكر الناس في العبودية ، يفكر الكثيرون في أن يكونوا مقيدين ومعصوبي الأعين .هناك العديد من الأصفاد الانفصالية التي تحاكي الإحساس بالتقييد ، ولكن إذا بدأ شخص ما في الذعر ، فيمكنه الانفصال .لا يجب أن يشمل مفهوم معصوب العينين التقييد، لكنهما يسيران جنبا إلى جنب في الغالب.

الهدف من التقييد هو السماح لشريكك بالتحكم الكامل في جسمك ، ولديك ما يكفي من الثقة في شريكك لمعرفة أنك لن تتضرر .إنه استسلام كامل .خذني الآن

افعل ما تريد معي ، أو اخترق أي ثقب بأي شكل من الأشكال أو لا تخترق على الإطلاق ، هذا هو التشويق من عصب ، العينين وتقييدك هو أنك لا تعرف ما سيحدث ، ولا يمكنك مقاومة حدوثه أيضا .إذا قام شخص ما بتقييدك إلى رف غزل وأراد أن يدورك حتى تتقيأ ، فيمكنه ذلك .قد يفاجئونك

فقط بالسياط والجليد ، وهذه هي طبيعة الوحش ، ولا يعرفون
ما سيفعله شريكك ، وينتظرون بترقب.

Getting Tied Up

Atarse

الربط

*Now that we know the point is more about
building anticipation, when someone asks if you
want to get tied up, be aware that knot tying is a
specialty skill in bondage. It's not like tying your
shoes. It's a process that can literally take hours as
I personally experienced when a dominatrix training
me asked if I wanted to be tied up on stage right
before the club opened, and by the time they were
done, they club was closing, hours later.*

*There can be a whole crew of people tying up
one person, with each person having their own
specialty knot tying skills. Not everyone approaches
it the same way. There are many ways to tie up a
captive for sexual pleasure, depending on how you
prefer penetration.*

*Keep in mind, there's a difference between
being handcuffed, strapped to a rack, and tied up in*

bondage. *Some people opt for the fisticuffs. Zipties are cheap.*

Ahora que sabemos que el punto es más sobre la construcción de la anticipación, cuando alguien te pregunta si quieres atarte, ten en cuenta que atar nudos es una habilidad especial en la esclavitud. No es como atarse los zapatos. Es un proceso que literalmente puede tomar horas, como experimenté personalmente cuando una dominatrix que me entrenaba me preguntó si quería estar atado al escenario justo antes de que el club abriera, y para cuando terminaron, el club estaba cerrando, horas después.

Puede haber todo un equipo de personas atando a una persona, y cada persona tiene sus propias habilidades especializadas para atar nudos. No todos lo abordan de la misma manera. Hay muchas maneras de atar a un cautivo para el placer sexual, dependiendo de cómo prefiera la penetración.

Tenga en cuenta que hay una diferencia entre estar esposado, atado a un estante y atado en esclavitud. Algunas personas optan por los puños. Las cremalleras son baratas.

الآن بعد أن عرفنا أن النقطة تتعلق أكثر ببناء الترقب ، عندما يسألك شخص ما عما إذا كنت تريد أن تقيد ، كن على

دراية بأن ربط العقدة هو مهارة متخصصة في العبودية .انها
ليست مثل ربط حذائك .إنها عملية يمكن أن تستغرق حرفيا
ساعات كما اختبرت شخصيا عندما سألني أحد مدربي
دوميناتريكس عما إذا كنت أرغب في أن أكون مقيدا على
خشبة المسرح قبل افتتاح النادي مباشرة ، وبحلول الوقت
الذي انتهوا فيه ، كان النادي يغلق ، بعد ساعات.

يمكن أن يكون هناك طاقم كامل من الأشخاص الذين يربطون
شخصا واحدا ، حيث يمتلك كل شخص مهاراته الخاصة في
ربط العقدة .لا يقترب الجميع منه بنفس الطريقة .هناك
العديد من الطرق لربط الأسير من أجل المتعة الجنسية ،
اعتمادا على الطريقة التي تفضل بها الإيلاج.

ضع في اعتبارك أن هناك فرقا بين تقييد اليدين
وربطهما على رف وربطهما في العبودية .بعض الناس
يختارون القبضات .ربطات سحاب رخيصة.

Whip Me, Please

Látigo, por favor

سوط لي ، من فضلك

Bondage is actually about respect, so most
Master's demand their slaves to say please, thank
you and call them by either Sir or Madam,
depending. They like their slaves to beg to be beaten,
wanting to find the pleasure in pain, and many
slaves will purposely try to act "naughty," so they

may receive their "punishment." In actuality, the punishment is a little pain, followed by intense pleasure, so the yin with the yang, both together.

When people want to get whipped, while there is pain, be mindful of where marks are left. Most professional dominatrices will advise to keep whipping to the bottom like spanking a child, or on the back, being mindful of the kidney region, as that can be dangerous. These are areas that can be easily covered when in public.

While horse whips might be used, the variety of whips are vast and expensive, with surprisingly soft beaver fur and lamb skin leather offering pleasure with the sting of pain. Fur items can be used to tickling, followed by the sting of the leather whipping the skin. It's like having melting ice cream on top of a hot pie, both sensations at once, like hot candle wax and ice.

La esclavitud en realidad se trata de respeto, por lo que la mayoría de los Maestros exigen a sus esclavos que digan por favor, gracias y llámelos por Señor o Señora, dependiendo. Les gusta que sus esclavos pidan ser golpeados, queriendo encontrar el placer en el dolor, y muchos esclavos tratarán deliberadamente de actuar "traviesos", para que puedan recibir su "castigo". En realidad, el castigo es un poco de dolor, seguido de un intenso placer, por lo que el yin con el yang, ambos juntos.

Cuando las personas quieren ser azotadas, mientras hay dolor, tenga en cuenta dónde quedan las marcas. La mayoría de las dominatrices profesionales aconsejarán seguir azotando hasta el fondo como azotar a un niño, o en la espalda, teniendo en cuenta la región del riñón, ya que eso puede ser peligroso. Estas son áreas que se pueden cubrir fácilmente cuando están en público.

Si bien se pueden usar látigos de caballo, la variedad de látigos es vasta y costosa, con piel de castor sorprendentemente suave y cuero de piel de cordero que ofrece placer con la picadura del dolor. Los artículos de piel se pueden usar para hacer cosquillas, seguidos de la picadura del cuero que azota la piel. Es como tener un helado derretido encima de un pastel caliente, ambas sensaciones a la vez, como cera de vela caliente y hielo.

العبودية هي في الواقع عن الاحترام ، لذلك يطلب معظم السيد من عبيدهم أن يقولوا من فضلك ، شكرا لك والاتصال بهم إما من قبل سيدي أو سيدتي ، اعتمادا على ذلك. إنهم يحبون عبيدهم أن يتوسلوا للضرب ، ويريدون أن يجدوا المتعة في الألم ، وسيحاول العديد من العبيد عمدا التصرف المشاغب" ، حتى يتمكنوا من الحصول على" عقابهم "في" الواقع ، العقاب هو القليل من الألم ، تليها متعة شديدة ، لذلك الين مع يانغ ، كلاهما معا.

عندما يرغب الناس في التعرض للجلد ، بينما يكون هناك ألم ضع في اعتبارك أين تترك العلامات ينصح معظم ،

الدوميناتريس المحترفين بالاستمرار في الجلد إلى القاع مثل ، ضرب الطفل ، أو على الظهر ، مع مراعاة منطقة الكلى لأن ذلك يمكن أن يكون خطيرا. هذه هي المجالات التي يمكن تغطيتها بسهولة عندما تكون في الأماكن العامة.

في حين يمكن استخدام سياط الخيول ، فإن مجموعة متنوعة من السياط واسعة ومكلفة ، مع فرو القندس الناعم بشكل مدهش وجلد جلد الضأن الذي يوفر المتعة مع لدغة الألم. يمكن استخدام عناصر الفراء في الدغدغة ، تليها لدغة الجلد الذي يجلد الجلد. الأمر يشبه إذابة الآيس كريم فوق فطيرة ساخنة ، وكلا الأحاسيس في وقت واحد ، مثل شمع الشموع الساخنة والثلج.

Shock Me, Please

Escúyame, por favor

صدمتني ، من فضلك

Being shocked in the world of bondage is not simply seeing or doing something outlandish, but it literally can refer to electrical shock. At low voltages, electrical currents running through a poked wheel on the skin feels like ants marching on the flesh. You don't have to be like Uncle Fester and run so high of a voltage that you're powering lightbulbs in your mouth.

Low voltage stimulation is merely different sensations on the flesh. There's a kit with different attachments that create different feelings when it touches your skin, and that sensation can intensify to an entirely different sensation when the voltage is cranked up a little too high. Again, it's finding your own personal threshold of how much is too much?

Keep in mind, if you or your partner have piercings, that metal is a conductor, so electrical stimulation on metal like piercings can intensify to the point of causing burns. Always be mindful of nearby conductors. Obviously, most importantly, be mindful of water, as water and electricity do not mix.

Ser impactado en el mundo de la esclavitud no es simplemente ver o hacer algo extravagante, sino que literalmente puede referirse a una descarga eléctrica. A bajos voltajes, las corrientes eléctricas que corren a través de una rueda pinchada en la piel se sienten como hormigas marchando sobre la carne. No tienes que ser como el tío Fester y correr tan alto de un voltaje que estás alimentando bombillas en tu boca.

La estimulación de bajo voltaje es simplemente sensaciones diferentes en la carne. Hay un kit con diferentes accesorios que crean diferentes sensaciones cuando toca su piel, y esa sensación puede intensificarse a una sensación completamente

diferente cuando el voltaje se eleva un poco
demasiado alto. Una vez más, ¿es encontrar su
propio umbral personal de cuánto es demasiado?

إن الصدمة في عالم العبودية ليست مجرد رؤية أو القيام
بشيء غريب ، ولكنها يمكن أن تشير حرفيا إلى صدمة
كهربائية .في الفولتية المنخفضة ، تبدو التيارات الكهربائية
التي تمر عبر عجلة ممزقة على الجلد وكأنها نمل يسير على
الجسد .ليس عليك أن تكون مثل العم فيستر وأن تعمل بجهد
عال لدرجة أنك تقوم بتشغيل المصابيح الكهربائية في فمك.

تحفيز الجهد المنخفض هو مجرد أحاسيس مختلفة على
الجسد .هناك مجموعة مع مرفقات مختلفة تخلق مشاعر
مختلفة عندما تلمس بشرتك ، ويمكن أن يكثف هذا الإحساس
إلى إحساس مختلف تماما عندما يتم رفع الجهد إلى أعلى
قليلا .مرة أخرى ، إنها تجد عتبة شخصية خاصة بك كم هو
أكثر من اللازم؟

Having Safe Word

Tener una palabra Segura

وجود كلمة آمنة

As bondage is about learning your own
personal limits with your partner, it is very
important that both of you have a safe word.

When having sex, especially during role play, no can really mean yes, and signals can get confused. Therefore, a safe word is something that has nothing to do with whatever role you are playing, such as "banana," and that word is said when that person is not feeling comfortable.

A safe word is a word that means stop. It's like saying "uncle" when rough-housing as a kid. It means that you are being too rough and to stop.

Safe words vary from person to person, but be sure that partner know each other's safe word before the bondage even starts. That way, there's no confusion if someone says "stop" when they mean "keep going," just because they are role playing a game, such as playing a victim part. An example of this might be a burglar role play where one partner act as if they are breaking into the house to take advantage of the other partner.

Como la esclavitud se trata de aprender sus propios límites personales con su pareja, es muy importante que ambos tengan una palabra segura. Al tener relaciones sexuales, especialmente durante el juego de roles, no puede significar realmente que sí, y las señales pueden confundirse. Por lo tanto, una palabra segura es algo que no tiene nada que ver con cualquier papel que esté desempeñando, como "plátano", y esa palabra se dice cuando esa persona no se siente cómoda.

Una palabra segura es una palabra que significa detener. Es como decir "tío" cuando se trata de un niño. Significa que estás siendo demasiado rudo y para detenerte.

Las palabras seguras varían de persona a persona, pero asegúrese de que la pareja conozca la palabra segura del otro antes de que comience la esclavitud. De esa manera, no hay confusión si alguien dice "detente" cuando quiere decir "sigue adelante", solo porque está jugando un juego de rol, como interpretar un papel de víctima. Un ejemplo de esto podría ser un juego de roles de ladrón en el que un compañero actúa como si estuviera irrumpiendo en la casa para aprovecharse del otro compañero.

نظرا لأن العبودية تدور حول تعلم حدودك الشخصية مع شريكك ، فمن المهم جدا أن يكون لدى كل منكما كلمة آمنة. عند ممارسة الجنس ، خاصة أثناء لعب الأدوار ، لا يمكن أن تعني نعم حقا ، ويمكن أن يتم الخلط بين الإشارات. لذلك فإن الكلمة الآمنة هي شيء لا علاقة له بأي دور تلعبه ، مثل

الموز "، وتقال هذه الكلمة عندما لا يشعر هذا الشخص
بالراحة.

الكلمة الآمنة هي كلمة تعني التوقف. انها مثل قول
"عم" عندما السكن الخشن عندما كنت طفلا. هذا يعني أنك
خشن للغاية ولا يمكنك التوقف.

تختلف الكلمات الآمنة من شخص لآخر، ولكن تأكد
من أن الشريك يعرف الكلمة الآمنة لبعضه البعض قبل أن
تبدأ العبودية. بهذه الطريقة، لا يوجد أي التباس إذا قال
شخص ما "توقف" عندما يعني "الاستمرار"، لمجرد أنه
يلعب دورا في لعبة، مثل لعب دور الضحية. مثال على ذلك
قد يكون لعب دور اللص حيث يتصرف أحد الشركاء كما لو
كان يقتحم المنزل للاستفادة من الشريك الآخر.

On Genital Piercings

Sobre los piercings genitales

على الثقوب التناسلية

*Personally, I maxxed out at ten vaginal
piercings, so I can only tell you what I know
personally to be true. No, not all piercings result in
some amazing pleasure. Yes, they can get caught at
inopportune moments and hurt when they get
yanked into a zipper unexpectedly.*

Be careful of tongue rings doing oral on a person with genital piercings, as they can and will get caught. I think of piercings as being like a bee sting, where it hurts momentarily, but it heals faster than people would think, especially since the genitals tend to be warm and moist. Yes, you will have to take them out for medical reasons, such as when getting an x-ray, as metal shows up.

People do not always get genital piercings for pleasure, as I got mine to be more like a built-in chastity belt, an excuse to not have sex. So, don't merely assume that a person is a whore if they have a genital piercing, as it may be completely to the contrary. The psychological reasons being body art often has more to do with being able to control an external pain when you cannot control an internal pain, so reasons highly vary.

Personalmente, llegué a diez piercings vaginales, así que solo puedo decirte lo que personalmente sé que es cierto. No, no todos los piercings resultan en un placer increíble. Sí, pueden quedar atrapados en momentos inoportunos y lastimarse cuando son tirados en una cremallera inesperadamente.

Tenga cuidado con los anillos de la lengua que se hacen oralmente en una persona con piercings genitales, ya que pueden y serán atrapados. Pienso en los piercings como una picadura de abeja, donde duele momentáneamente, pero se cura más rápido de lo que la gente pensaría, especialmente porque los genitales tienden a ser cálidos y húmedos. Sí, tendrá que sacarlos por razones médicas, como cuando se hace una radiografía, ya que aparece el metal.

La gente no siempre se hace piercings genitales por placer, ya que conseguí que el mío fuera más como un cinturón de castidad incorporado, una excusa para no tener relaciones sexuales. Por lo tanto, no asuma simplemente que una persona es una puta si tiene un piercing genital, ya que puede ser completamente al contrario. Las razones psicológicas por las que el arte corporal a menudo tiene más que ver con poder controlar un dolor externo cuando no se puede controlar un dolor interno, por lo que las razones varían mucho.

أنا شخصيا ، وصلت إلى عشرة ثقوب مهبلية ، لذلك لا يسعني إلا أن أخبرك بما أعرفه شخصيا ليكون صحيحا. لا ، ليست كل الثقوب تؤدي إلى بعض المتعة المدهشة. نعم يمكن أن يتم القبض عليهم في لحظات غير مناسبة ويتألمون عندما يتم سحبهم إلى سحاب بشكل غير متوقع.

كن حذرا من حلقات اللسان التي تحدث عن طريق الفم على شخص مصاب بثقوب الأعضاء التناسلية ، حيث يمكن أن يتم القبض عليهم وسوف يتم القبض عليهم. أفكر في الثقوب على أنها مثل لدغة النحل ، حيث تؤلم للحظات لكنها تشفى بشكل أسرع مما يعتقد الناس ، خاصة وأن

، الأعضاء التناسلية تميل إلى أن تكون دافئة ورطبة. نعم
سيتعين عليك إخراجها لأسباب طبية ، مثل عند الحصول
على أشعة سينية ، حيث يظهر المعدن.

لا يحصل الناس دائما على ثقوب الأعضاء التناسلية
من أجل المتعة ، حيث حصلت على أن أكون أشبه بحزام عفة
مدمج ، وهو عذر لعدم ممارسة الجنس. لذا ، لا تفترض فقط
، أن الشخص عاهرة إذا كان لديه ثقب في الأعضاء التناسلية
لأنه قد يكون على العكس تماما. غالبا ما تكون الأسباب
النفسية لفن الجسد أكثر ارتباطا بالقدرة على التحكم في الألم
الخارجي عندما لا يمكنك التحكم في ألم داخلي ، لذلك تختلف
الأسباب اختلافا كبيرا.

On Tantric Sex

Sobre el sexo tántrico

على جنس التانترا

Trantic sex is about using each other's life
force. Yes, it's about being in tune with each other,
breathing at the same time with each other, and
ultimately, trying to climax at the same time with
each other. It's also about capturing the life force of
the young to the old.

When I dated a Syrian guy who was older
than me, one of the first things he did was make me
read a book on tantric sex, so I understood how it

truly worked. When there's an age difference, it's like the older partner is sharing the energy of the younger partner, consuming their essence during sex, but ultimately at mutual climax. That's how you know you're in tune with each other, when you can actually climax at the same time together, and one of the only partners that nearly every time did that was my celestial opposite: May 3 and November 3, North and South, polar opposites, Taurus and Scorpio.

It's the give and take. Youth gives to the elder. There's a lot more to it than that, and I would highly advise doing your own research, but it's a great way to learn to be in tune with yourself, as well as your partner.

El sexo trantico se trata de usar la fuerza vital del otro. Sí, se trata de estar en sintonía el uno con el otro, respirar al mismo tiempo entre sí y, en última instancia, tratar de llegar al clímax al mismo tiempo entre sí. También se trata de capturar la fuerza vital de los jóvenes a los viejos.

Cuando salí con un hombre sirio que era mayor que yo, una de las primeras cosas que hizo fue hacerme leer un libro sobre sexo tántrico, así que entendí cómo funcionaba realmente. Cuando hay una diferencia de edad, es como si la pareja mayor estuviera compartiendo la energía de la pareja más joven, consumiendo su esencia durante el sexo, pero en última instancia en el clímax mutuo. Así es como sabes que estás en sintonía el uno con el otro, cuando en realidad puedes llegar al clímax al mismo tiempo juntos, y uno de los únicos socios que casi siempre lo hizo fue mi opuesto celestial: 3 de mayo y 3 de noviembre, Norte y Sur, polos opuestos, Tauro y Escorpio.

Es el toma y daca. La juventud da al anciano. Hay mucho más que eso, y le recomiendo encarecidamente que haga su propia investigación, pero es una excelente manera de aprender a estar en sintonía consigo mismo, así como con su pareja.

الجنس التكرانتي يدور حول استخدام قوة حياة بعضهم البعض. نعم ، يتعلق الأمر بالتناغم مع بعضنا البعض ، والتنفس في نفس الوقت مع بعضنا البعض ، وفي النهاية محاولة الذروة في نفس الوقت مع بعضنا البعض. يتعلق الأمر أيضا بالتقاط قوة حياة الصغار إلى الكبار.

عندما واعدت رجلا سوريا أكبر مني سنا، كان أحد أول الأشياء التي قام بها هو جعلني أقرأ كتابا عن جنس التانترا، لذلك فهمت كيف كان يعمل حقا. عندما يكون هناك فارق في العمر ، يبدو الأمر كما لو أن الشريك الأكبر سنا يشارك طاقة الشريك الأصغر سنا، ويستهلك جوهره أثناء ممارسة الجنس ، ولكن في النهاية في ذروة متبادلة.

هذه هي الطريقة التي تعرف بها أنك متناغم مع بعضكما البعض ، عندما يمكنك في الواقع الذروة في نفس الوقت معا وكان أحد الشركاء الوحيدين الذين فعلوا ذلك في كل مرة

تقريبا هو نقيضي السماوي 3: مايو و 3 نوفمبر ، الشمـال والجنوب ، الأضداد القطبية ، الثور والعقرب.

إنه الأخذ والعطاء .الشباب يعطي للشيخ .هناك ما هو أكثر من ذلك بكثير ، وأنصح بشدة بإجراء أبحاثك الخاصة ، ولكنها طريقة رائعة لتعلم أن تكون متناغما مع نفسك ، وكذلك شريكك.

Having Mutual Orgasm

Tener orgasmo mutuo

وجود هزة الجماع المتبادلة

You both have to work at having a mutual orgasm, but it's best when it happens naturally. For both partners to orgasm simultaneously, it can help to try to breathe at the same time, in synch with each other. Getting into the same rhythm, if you will, helps timing.

Hips moving at the same time, do not try to focus too hard on being exactly inhale exhale at the same time, as if you focus on one thing, you may distract from another, so it's very much about be there now in bed. If one speeds up, the other speeds up, so it's mimicking a bit. If you can see your partner letting go, try to let go at the same time, relax, and enjoy the moment together.

Do what your partner does when your partner does it, so if one slows up, the other slows up. If one intensifies, the other's intensity should increase as well. They key is to find that perfect rhythm together as one.

Ambos tienen que trabajar para tener un orgasmo mutuo, pero es mejor cuando sucede naturalmente. Para que ambos miembros de la pareja tengan un orgasmo simultáneamente, puede ser útil tratar de respirar al mismo tiempo, en sincronía entre sí. Entrar en el mismo ritmo, si se quiere, ayuda al tiempo.

Las caderas se mueven al mismo tiempo, no trates de concentrarte demasiado en estar exactamente inhalando exhala al mismo tiempo, ya que si te enfocas en una cosa, puedes distraerte de otra, por lo que se trata mucho de estar allí ahora en la cama. Si uno acelera, el otro se acelera, por lo que está imitando un poco. Si puedes ver a tu pareja soltándose, trata de dejarlo ir al mismo tiempo, relájate y disfruta del momento juntos.

Haz lo que tu pareja hace cuando tu pareja lo hace, así que si uno se ralentiza, el otro se ralentiza. Si uno se intensifica, la intensidad del otro también debería aumentar. La clave es encontrar ese ritmo perfecto juntos como uno solo.

كلاكما يجب أن يعمل على الحصول على هزة الجماع المتبادلة ، ولكن من الأفضل عندما يحدث ذلك بشكل طبيعي. بالنسبة لكلا الشريكين للوصول إلى النشوة الجنسية في وقت واحد ، ، يمكن أن يساعد في محاولة التنفس في نفس الوقت بالتزامن مع بعضهما البعض. الدخول في نفس الإيقاع ، إذا صح التعبير ، يساعد على التوقيت.

تتحرك الوركين في نفس الوقت ، لا تحاول التركيز بشدة على استنشاق الزفير بالضبط في نفس الوقت ، كما لو كنت تركز على شيء واحد ، فقد تشتت انتباهك عن شيء آخر ، لذلك يتعلق الأمر كثيرا بالتواجد الآن في السرير. إذا تسارع أحدهما ، فإن الآخر يسرع ، لذلك فهو يحاكي قليلا. إذا كنت تستطيع رؤية شريكك يتخلى عنه ، فحاول تركه في نفس الوقت ، والاسترخاء ، والاستمتاع باللحظة معا.

افعل ما يفعله شريكك عندما يفعل شريكك ذلك ، لذلك إذا تباطأ أحدهما ، فإن الآخر يتباطأ. إذا اشتد أحدهما ، فيجب أن تزداد شدة الآخر أيضا. المفتاح هو العثور على هذا الإيقاع المثالي معا كواحد.

All About Anal

Todo sobre Anal

كل شيء عن الشرج

Do not just jam it in all at once without lube. That's one way to send a partner scurrying across the bed. Be considerate, go slow, especially for a first time, and use lubrication to try to avoid anal tearing, bleeding.

Stimulate the front side to make the back side relax, especially with women, as the pelvis needs to relax. Stimulating the clitoris is very important with women, especially the first timers. Do not take the hand off the clit, just keep rubbing in a circular motion, or use a dildo.

With men, a reach around can be a great addition to anal stimulation. With women, most important, never pull out of the anus and go into the vagina, as that will create urinary infections, and nobody likes to piss blood. Regardless of the gender, oral preferences for anal can vary, as some like gentle flickers, while others prefer the ferocious style of eating that ass like you're starving.

For Foot Fetishes

Para fetiches de pies

لأوثان القدم

Not everyone has a foot fetish, so respect when people do not want to have their feet touched, as for some people it is simply too sensitive an area for stimulation. Some people are reluctant to explore their feet as an area of stimulation, but for years, people have touted how simple foot massages can increase circulation. This alone is a reason to try it.

Massaging the feet is one thing that is more than meets the eye, as there are charts pointing to which part of the foot correlates with other parts of the body. There's a lot of learn about the subject. In general, the pads of the feet underneath the toes, as well as the arch of the foot and heel, are great places to start for even the most basic foot massages.

During sex, sucking on the foot can heighten arousal, adding to the sexual stimulation, increasing orgasm. Again, some people are more into this than others, so talk to your lover. Sometimes, an attempt at surprising someone by sucking their foot can result in a kick to the face as a knee jerk reaction, so be warned, it may be best to go slow to check their reaction to that kind of stimulation and be prepared.

No todo el mundo tiene un fetiche en los pies, así que respeta cuando las personas no quieren que les toquen los pies, ya que para algunas personas es simplemente un área demasiado sensible para la estimulación. Algunas personas son reacias a explorar sus pies como un área de estimulación, pero durante años, las personas han promocionado cómo los masajes simples de pies pueden aumentar la circulación. Esto solo es una razón para probarlo.

Masajear los pies es una cosa que es más de lo
que parece, ya que hay gráficos que apuntan a qué
parte del pie se correlaciona con otras partes del
cuerpo. Hay mucho que aprender sobre el tema. En
general, las almohadillas de los pies debajo de los
dedos de los pies, así como el arco del pie y el talón,
son excelentes lugares para comenzar incluso para
los masajes de pies más básicos.

Durante el sexo, chupar el pie puede
aumentar la excitación, lo que aumenta la
estimulación sexual, aumentando el orgasmo. Una
vez más, algunas personas están más interesadas en
esto que otras, así que habla con tu amante. A veces,
un intento de sorprender a alguien chupándole el pie
puede resultar en una patada en la cara como una
reacción instintiva, así que ten cuidado, puede ser
mejor ir despacio para comprobar su reacción a ese
tipo de estimulación y estar preparado.

ليس كل شخص لديه صنم القدم ، لذلك احترم عندما لا يرغب
الناس في لمس أقدامهم ، كما هو الحال بالنسبة لبعض الناس
فهي ببساطة منطقة حساسة للغاية للتحفيز   .بعض الناس ،
يترددون في استكشاف أقدامهم كمنطقة للتحفيز ، ولكن
لسنوات ، وصف الناس كيف يمكن لتدليك القدم البسيط أن
يزيد من الدورة الدموية .هذا وحده هو سبب لتجربته.

تدليك القدمين هو شيء واحد أكثر مما تراه العين ، حيث
توجد مخططات تشير إلى أي جزء من القدم يرتبط بأجزاء
أخرى من الجسم .هناك الكثير من التعلم حول هذا

الموضوع .بشكل عام ، تعد منصات القدمين تحت أصابع
القدم ، وكذلك قوس القدم والكعب ، أماكن رائعة للبدء حتى
في تدليك القدم الأساسي.

أثناء ممارسة الجنس ، يمكن أن يؤدي مص القدم
إلى زيادة الإثارة ، مما يزيد من التحفيز الجنسي ، مما يزيد
من النشوة الجنسية .مرة أخرى ، بعض الناس أكثر اهتماما
بهذا من غيرهم ، لذا تحدث إلى حبيبك .في بعض الأحيان ،
يمكن أن تؤدي محاولة مفاجأة شخص ما عن طريق مص
قدمه إلى ركلة على الوجه كرد فعل على الركبة ، لذلك كن
حذرا ، قد يكون من الأفضل أن تسير ببطء للتحقق من رد
فعله على هذا النوع من التحفيز وتكون مستعدا.

On Hair Pulling

Sobre el tirón del cabello

على شد الشعر

*As someone with long hair, I can honestly
say I do not always like to have my hair pulled. For
me, my concern is more for injuring the neck, as some
people simply get carried away and are too heavy-
handed. If it's a playful tug, that's one thing, but I
do not want to have globs of hair missing from my
head, as bald patches are never really seen as sexy.*

*Some people like it. Not everyone. Be
mindful that not everyone likes the same thing.*

If someone is into it, wrapping the hair around the hand can be a good way to get control. Don't pull out individual strands. It should feel good, enhancing stimulation, not hurting the neck.

Como alguien con el pelo largo, puedo decir honestamente que no siempre me gusta que me tiren del pelo. Para mí, mi preocupación es más por lesionar el cuello, ya que algunas personas simplemente se dejan llevar y son demasiado pesadas. Si es un tirón juguetón, eso es una cosa, pero no quiero que me falten gotas de pelo en la cabeza, ya que los parches de calvicie nunca se ven realmente como sexys.

A algunas personas les gusta. No todos. Ten en cuenta que no a todo el mundo le gusta lo mismo.

Si a alguien le gusta, envolver el cabello alrededor de la mano puede ser una buena manera de obtener el control. No saque hebras individuales. Debe sentirse bien, mejorando la estimulación, no lastimando el cuello.

كشخص ذو شعر طويل ، يمكنني أن أقول بصراحة أنني لا أحب دائما أن أسحب شعري .بالنسبة لي ، فإن قلقي أكثر من إصابة الرقبة ، لأن بعض الناس ببساطة ينجرفون بعيدا ويكونون ثقيلي اليدين .إذا كان الأمر يتعلق بشد لعوب ، فهذا شيء واحد ، لكنني لا أريد أن يكون لدي كرات من الشعر

مفقودة من رأسي ، حيث لا ينظر إلى البقع الصلعاء أبدا على أنها مثيرة.

بعض الناس يحبون ذلك. ليس الجميع. ضع في اعتبارك أنه ليس كل شخص يحب نفس الشيء.

إذا كان شخص ما في ذلك ، فإن لف الشعر حول اليد يمكن أن يكون وسيلة جيدة للسيطرة عليه. لا تسحب خيوطا فردية. يجب أن تشعر بالرضا ، وتعزيز التحفيز ، وعدم إيذاء الرقبة.

Breasts Are Tender

Los senos están sensibles

الثديان طريان

While some people like nipple stimulation, keep in mind that breasts are tender. Bruised breasts can result in lumps that can turn into medical issues. Remember this when you're getting rough in the bed, as medical bills are never sexy.

Different people have different tolerances. Sometimes, guys have more sensitive nipples than women, believe it or not. Some say since men typically have smaller breasts with less fat blocking the nerve endings that this could be why perhaps.

Having seen huge biker dudes straight up pass out when getting their nipples pierced supports this claim. Be mindful when stimulating sensitive areas, as there can be a fine line between pleasure and pain. Always respect your partner's boundaries.

Si bien a algunas personas les gusta la estimulación del pezón, tenga en cuenta que los senos son sensibles. Los senos magullados pueden provocar bultos que pueden convertirse en problemas médicos. Recuerde esto cuando se ponga áspero en la cama, ya que las facturas médicas nunca son sexys.

Diferentes personas tienen diferentes tolerancias. A veces, los hombres tienen pezones más sensibles que las mujeres, lo creas o no. Algunos dicen que dado que los hombres suelen tener senos más pequeños con menos grasa que bloquea las terminaciones nerviosas, esto podría ser la razón tal vez.

Haber visto a enormes tipos moteros desmayarse al perforarse los pezones apoya esta afirmación. Tenga en cuenta al estimular áreas sensibles, ya que puede haber una delgada línea entre el placer y el dolor. Respeta siempre los límites de tu pareja.

في حين أن بعض الناس يحبون تحفيز الحلمة ، ضع في اعتبارك أن الثديين طريان .يمكن أن يؤدي الثدي المصاب بكدمات إلى كتل يمكن أن تتحول إلى مشاكل طبية .تذكر هذا عندما تصبح خشنا في السرير ، لأن الفواتير الطبية ليست مثيرة أبدا.

الأشخاص المختلفون لديهم تسامح مختلف .في بعض الأحيان ، يكون لدى الرجال حلمات أكثر حساسية من النساء ، صدق أو لا تصدق .يقول البعض بما أن الرجال عادة ما يكون لديهم ثديين أصغر مع كمية أقل من الدهون التي تسد النهايات العصبية ، فقد يكون هذا هو السبب في ذلك.

بعد أن رأيت الرجال راكبي الدراجات الضخمة على التوالي يمررون عند ثقب حلماتهم يدعم هذا الادعاء .كن حذرا عند تحفيز المناطق الحساسة ، حيث يمكن أن يكون هناك خط رفيع بين المتعة والألم .احترم دائما حدود شريكك.

Disclaimer

Renuncia

اخلاء المسؤوليه

A translation program was used for the Spanish and Arabic languages in this book, so forgive any errors from the translation program.

Se utilizó un programa de traducción para los idiomas español y árabe en este libro, así que perdona cualquier error del programa de traducción.

تم استخدام برنامج ترجمة للغتين الإسبانية والعربية
في هذا الكتاب ، لذا اغفر أي أخطاء من برنامج الترجمة.

*This book is in no way, shape, or form advice
from any sort of licensed professional of any kind.
This was written from a common sense and
experience perspective. Do not hate me if the advice
does not work out in your favor; pick and choose
what works best for you, as it's your life.*

*Este libro no es de ninguna manera, forma o
forma de consejo de ningún tipo de profesional con
licencia de ningún tipo. Esto fue escrito desde una
perspectiva de sentido común y experiencia. No me
odies si el consejo no funciona a tu favor; elige lo que
funciona mejor para ti, ya que es tu vida.*

هذا الكتاب ليس بأي حال من الأحوال أو شكل أو
شكل نصيحة من أي نوع من المهنيين المرخصين من أي
نوع. وقد كتب هذا من منظور الحس السليم والخبرة. لا
تكرهني إذا لم تنجح النصيحة في صالحك. اختر واختر ما
يناسبك ، لأنها حياتك.

More by Marisa

Más de Marisa

المزيد من ماريسا

For more by Marisa, visit
www.outlandishwriter.com,
www.lulu.com/spotlight/thorisaz, follow her on
Twitter @Booksnbling, or on Instagram @Thorisaz

Para obtener más información sobre Marisa, visite
www.outlandishwriter.com,
www.lulu.com/spotlight/thorisaz, sígala en Twitter
@Booksnbling o en Instagram @Thorisaz

لمعرفة المزيد من ماريسا، تفضل بزيارة
أو www.outlandishwriter.com
أو تابعها على تويتر www.lulu.com/spotlight/thorisaz
@Booksnbling أو على إنستغرام @Thorisaz